Educating Health Professionals
in Low-Resource Countries

A Global Approach

Joyce P. Murray, EdD, RN, FAAN, became director of The Carter Center's Ethiopia Public Health Training Initiative in 2002, to meet the educational and training needs of staff at over 500 new health centers in Ethiopia. A past president of the National League for Nursing, she holds a professorship in nursing at Emory University. Having worked extensively in mental health nursing, curriculum development, leadership, and service, she brings to the developing country health science education milieu a broad portfolio of experience in nursing practice, education, and public health. Dr. Murray is one of the principal originators of the educational materials described in this book. She is frequently published in the nursing literature, appears at major nursing meetings internationally, and is a Fellow of the American Academy of Nursing.

Anna Frances Z. Wenger, PhD, RN, FAAN, is Professor and Director Emeritus of Nursing at Goshen College, Goshen, Indiana, where she was codirector of study-service terms in Haiti, Nicaragua, and Germany. She lived and worked in Ghana, West Africa, for 2 years. Dr. Wenger is a past associate professor of nursing at the Nell Hodgson Woodruff School of Nursing at Emory University, Atlanta, Georgia, and continues as Senior Scholar, Interfaith Health Program, Rollins School of Public Health, Emory University. As faculty consultant to the Ethiopia Public Health Initiative, she is one of the principal originators of the educational materials described in this book. She has published numerous peer-reviewed journal articles and has contributed to several books on transcultural nursing. She is past president of the Transcultural Nursing Society, a member of the Transcultural Nursing Scholars, and a Fellow of the American Academy of Nursing.

Elizabeth A. Downes, MPH, MSN, APRN-BC, is an assistant clinical professor at the Nell Hodgson Woodruff School of Nursing at Emory University, Atlanta, Georgia, and a family nurse practitioner with more than 20 years of experience in international health. She is a consultant to the Ethiopia Public Health Training Initiative and has worked with the World Health Organization's regional office in the Western Pacific to develop and implement an educational program for the preparation of nurse practitioners. Ms. Downes is one of the principal originators of the educational materials described in this book. She also has worked with various nongovernmental organizations, including the International Rescue Committee, Save the Children, CARE, and Health Volunteers Overseas. Ms. Downes also has worked directly with governmental agencies, such as the Ministry of Health in Mozambique, the U.S. Agency for International Development, and the Peace Corps.

Shelly B. Terrazas, MBA, MS, is assistant director of the Ethiopia Public Health Training Initiative (EPHTI) and Mental Health Liberia Program at The Carter Center in Atlanta, Georgia. With 10 years' experience in international research and development work, Ms. Terrazas assists health sciences universities in Ethiopia to develop curricula, teaching materials, faculty skills, and campus learning environments to enhance the quality of health education in the country, while managing the day-to-day operations of the EPHTI.

Educating Health Professionals in Low-Resource Countries

A Global Approach

Joyce P. Murray, EdD, RN, FAAN
Anna Frances Z. Wenger, PhD, RN, FAAN
Elizabeth A. Downes, MPH, MSN, APRN-BC
Shelly B. Terrazas, MBA, MS

THE
CARTER CENTER

SPRINGER PUBLISHING COMPANY
NEW YORK

Springer Publishing Company, LLC
11 West 42nd Street
New York, NY 10036
www.springerpub.com

Acquisitions Editor: Allan Graubard
Production Editor: Gayle Lee
Cover Design: David Levy
Project Manager: Vanavan Jayaraman
Composition: S4Carlisle Publishing Services

ISBN: 978-0-8261-3257-4
E-book ISBN: 978-0-8261-3258-1

10 11 12 13/ 5 4 3 2 1

The author and the publisher of this Work have made every effort to use sources believed to be reliable to provide information that is accurate and compatible with the standards generally accepted at the time of publication. Because medical science is continually advancing, our knowledge base continues to expand. Therefore, as new information becomes available, changes in procedures become necessary. We recommend that the reader always consult current research and specific institutional policies before performing any clinical procedure. The author and publisher shall not be liable for any special, consequential, or exemplary damages resulting, in whole or in part, from the readers' use of, or reliance on, the information contained in this book. The publisher has no responsibility for the persistence or accuracy of URLs for external or third-party Internet Web sites referred to in this publication and does not guarantee that any content on such Web sites is, or will remain, accurate or appropriate.

Library of Congress Cataloging-in-Publication Data

Educating health professionals in low-resource countries :
  a global approach / Joyce P. Murray . . . [et al.].
    p. cm.
  ISBN 978-0-8261-3257-4
 1. Medical education—Developing countries.   I. Murray, Joyce P.
  R737.E2855 2011
  610.71'11724—dc22

                                                         2010030641

Special discounts on bulk quantities of our books are available to corporations, professional associations, pharmaceutical companies, health care organizations, and other qualifying groups.

If you are interested in a custom book, including chapters from more than one of our titles, we can provide that service as well.

For details, please contact:
Special Sales Department, Springer Publishing Company, LLC
11 West 42nd Street, 15th Floor, New York, NY 10036-8002
Phone: 877-687-7476 or 212-431-4370; Fax: 212-941-7842
Email: sales@springerpub.com

Printed in the United States of America by Hamilton Printing.

This book is designed to engage health science teachers and students in the process of teaching and learning, specifically about the philosophy, methods, and strategies used in the education of health care providers. It was written for the preparation of teachers in pre-service and in-service educational settings, especially those in low-resource countries and environments where material, technological, and electronic resources are often limited. Persons who will find this book most helpful are teachers, experienced and new, who are providing or will provide health science education in challenging settings. The evidence base for this book derives from ten years of teaching learning workshops with health sciences faculty from seven Ethiopian universities, as part of the Ethiopia Public Heath Training Initiative sponsored by The Carter Center in Atlanta, Georgia, USA, and the Ministries of Health and Education of Ethiopia.

About The Carter Center

"Waging Peace. Fighting Disease. Building Hope."

A not-for-profit, nongovernmental organization, The Carter Center has helped to improve life for people in more than 70 countries by resolving conflicts; advancing democracy, human rights, and economic opportunity; preventing diseases; improving mental health care; and teaching farmers in developing nations to increase crop production. The Carter Center was founded in 1982 by former U.S. President Jimmy Carter and his wife, Rosalynn, in partnership with Emory University, to advance peace and health worldwide. Please visit www.cartercenter.org to learn more about The Carter Center.

About the Ethiopia Public Health Training Initiative

Because the biggest hurdle to better health in Ethiopia is the lack of access to health personnel, the mission of the Ethiopia Public Health Training Initiative (EPHTI) is to build a team of qualified health care workers across the country, especially in underserved rural populations. Launched in 1997, the EPHTI aims to improve the quality of pre-service training to health science professionals within Ethiopia through a partnership between the Ethiopian government, The Carter Center, the Ethiopia Ministry of Education, the Ethiopia Ministry of Health, and seven Ethiopian higher education universities. Improved training results in improved health care delivery for the entire population. The underlying assumption of the program is that Ethiopians know the best way to deliver public health care to Ethiopians.

To the faculty participants of the 13 teaching learning workshops held by the Ethiopia Public Health Training Initiative of The Carter Center from Addis Ababa University, Defense College of Health Sciences, University of Gondar, Hawassa University, Haramaya University, Jimma University, and Mekelle University. Your dedication to improving the education of health professionals in your country, and thus Ethiopia's future, has been an inspiration.

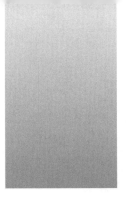

Contents

Foreword   *xiii*
Preface   *xvii*
Acknowledgments   *xix*
Introduction   *xxi*

1. What Is Teaching? What Is Learning? What Is Active Teaching Learning?   *1*

2. Theories and Research Supporting Active Teaching Learning Strategies   *17*

3. Understanding the Learner   *29*

4. Teaching in Classroom Settings   *51*

5. Tools for Teaching   *67*

6. Interactive Group Learning: The Use of Case Studies, Role Play, Simulations, Problem-Based Learning, and Service–Learning   *99*

7. Teaching in a Clinical Setting   *123*

8. Evaluation and Assessment   *137*

9. The Teacher as Leader, Role Model, and Mentor   *151*

10. Training Health Care Professionals in Low-Resource Environments: Applying Active Teaching Learning Strategies in Ethiopia   *159*

Index   *173*

Foreword

As is often true in health science teaching institutions in many countries, especially developing ones, the Ethiopian setting suffers from a lack of instructors with appropriate pedagogical skills. The selection of teachers for institutions of higher education has primarily depended on applications submitted by candidates in response to an advertisement. Incentives such as staying in relatively urban settings where universities are located and the potential for getting further education have been the major attraction. One key criterion used has been grades earned upon graduation, which may not guarantee that one will be a good prospective teacher. As a result, an applicant for a teaching position, and therefore a recruit, may not be appropriate for the teaching profession.

In addition, the health field has been subject to the tradition in which a senior teacher serves as the only role model for junior teachers. Unfortunately, the prevailing approach was not student centered; instead, it has been teacher centered, with one-way communication. Furthermore, this long-standing tradition has been handed down from the older universities to the newly established ones through young graduates from the former who have been emulating their own professors. Even the little experience gained through teaching in the more geographically remote universities is not available for long, because most young instructors leave to obtain further education, and usually they do not return. The resulting high turnover of health science instructors in universities aggravates the situation.

In the 1990s, the Ethiopian government and The Carter Center considered ways of collaboration. Capacity building for developing human resources in the field of health education was identified as a priority. Ethiopia, just coming out of a long civil war, was striving to rehabilitate its health services. For this to happen, the shortage of human resources had to be addressed. The government established three new universities in addition to the existing three. The sudden doubling of universities meant an escalated need for instructors. In the face of this urgency there was no time for a careful, rigorous selection of new instructors, and whoever applied was accepted to teach. Although this did not necessarily mean all were poor instructors, it left much to be desired in terms of quality education. Such a lack of comprehensive minimum skill requirements for new health science instructors was one of the major needs that the new joint venture between the Ethiopian government and The Carter Center was meant to address. It was agreed that university instructors should receive training in teaching and clinical supervision skills. The shortage of adequate and relevant reference materials also required attention; hence, individual teachers would prepare their own materials, which meant there was a lot of variation from university to university. Moreover, the teaching learning environment needed enhancement through the provision of basic health science classroom equipment and teaching aids.

This scenario led to the creation of a partnership between the Ethiopian government and The Carter Center. Major financial support came from the U.S. Agency for International Development in 2000, with additional funding from others, including the David and Lucile Packard Foundation, which contributed to specific activities. The key strategy was to create the Ethiopia Public Health Training Initiative (EPHTI) to serve as the secretariat for a network of the five (later, seven) existing government universities that were to participate in the endeavor. The program used technical consultants from several universities, with Emory University as a key contributor, providing the director of the program in 2002 and leading the teaching workshops in the summer. The EPHTI network of universities was responsible for the joint planning of activities, a project budget, and assignment of specific tasks to member institutions. Instructors were trained in writing skills. Standardized teaching materials were developed locally, and thousands of copies were printed and distributed for use by all teaching institutions.

Emory University professors came to Ethiopia for 2-week annual workshops during which they gave pedagogical and clinical supervision skills training for instructors. The instructors who participated in these workshops would then return to their respective universities and give 5-day cascade teaching methodology courses on their campuses. An interesting extension of this process occurred when nonuniversity hospitals were recruited to provide preservice teaching, which meant service providers had to be trained in pedagogical skills by the university faculty. Overall, close to 4,000 teachers in universities and hospitals received the training provided by these annual 2-week workshops.

In terms of outcome and impact, we observed a rapid transformation of the Ethiopian health sciences teaching landscape by instilling the right skills and attitude in both the university faculty and nonteaching hospital settings. Feedback from faculty, students, and peers showed that instructors who received pedagogical training were much more effective than nontrained ones. This was also true for the same teacher before and after he or she received the Carter Center–assisted training. Teachers assigned by default felt a good fit with, and developed a lasting affection for, the profession. Some who were co-opted from service-providing facilities ended up being long-term preservice educators! Some instructors wished their past university professors who lacked such skills be offered the training.

I believe such capacity-building partnerships can serve as a model in other low-resource settings. I would like to recognize the great dedication of the Emory professors who have put the teaching learning experiences in Ethiopia into a resource that will serve as a guide for teaching skills training in other low-resource environments. The role of the EPHTI network, the Addis Ababa office staff, and the EPHTI council members has also been critical in project implementation and ensuring sustainability.

Hailu Yeneneh, MD, MSc, BSc
Resident Technical Advisor
The Carter Center-Assisted
Ethiopia Public Health
Training Initiative

Preface

My wife Rosalynn and I have been traveling to Ethiopia and to other developing nations for years, beginning when I was President. After my presidency, I returned to Ethiopia when the Derg regime was still in power and when Mengistu, the communist dictator, was oppressing the country. I knew Prime Minister Meles Zenawi quite well, long before he was able to get to Addis Ababa and overthrow the oppressive Derg regime. In 1989, he was successful and inherited 75 to 80 million constituents in one of the poorest nations on earth, with the highest incidence of blindness in the world. Since that time great progress has been made in many areas, but especially in the health sector. The Derg regime was overthrown just 2 years before then-acting Prime Minister Meles Zenawi and I began talking about the Ethiopia Public Health Training Initiative (EPHTI) program. An initial idea was to create a school of public health, because at that time none existed in Ethiopia. Later, we thought it might be beneficial to let the school of public health in Ethiopia cooperate with a major university in the United States, and it was no accident that we choose Emory University, because I have been a professor there since I was President. I have enjoyed teaching at Emory for 28 years. Since 1997, we've continued to work on the EPHTI program, but in the early stages of Ethiopia's new government it was difficult to get the interorganizational framework established. One of the greatest triumphs for EPHTI has been cooperation between the Ministry of Health and Ministry of Education. The Carter Center has programs in 35 different African nations, and we know how rare it is to get health and education ministries to cooperate as thoroughly and as enthusiastically as they have in Ethiopia.

In 1997, Ethiopia and The Carter Center formed the EPHTI team and invited members to come to The Carter Center in Atlanta, Georgia. During that meeting we changed our concept from a single school of public health to creating 500 community health centers around Ethiopia, because Prime Minister Zenawi felt that the services to be provided should be dispersed throughout the country, not just concentrated in the capital city. We established a mechanism that trains instructors and staff who then teach health students. Between 1997 and 2000, we depended on pedagogical and skill-based workshops to train these workers to staff the new health centers around Ethiopia. In the year 2000, we received funds from U.S.

Agency for International Development (USAID) and the David and Lucile Packard Foundation to embark on the EPHTI as a major project. Along with providing training in teaching-learning and service-learning, the EPHTI assisted the universities of Ethiopia in creating locally developed curricula for their health classrooms, as well as providing some of the materials needed to train health professionals (e.g., computers, anatomical models, reference books, and other teaching aids).

We were somewhat constrained by instructions from Prime Minister Zenawi and the Ministers to concentrate on diseases afflicting the Ethiopian people. At first there were 30 diseases identified to tackle, and The Carter Center agreed to work with Ethiopia to develop a complete training module for each of those diseases. That was in the early stages of this project. Since then we've completed those 30 modules and have expanded to almost 230 types of health learning materials created based on the Ethiopian context, so 230 analyses of diseases or health topics that afflict Ethiopia have been created and now can be used to teach Ethiopians how to provide health care within their own country. These curricula are posted on The Carter Center's Web site and are available at no cost to anyone who seeks them. In addition, through our own funds, and through contributions from other sources, more than $1 million worth of textbooks have been provided for the different public health schools now in Ethiopia. We've held 565 workshops, some in the capital, Addis Ababa, but mostly scattered all over the nation. These workshops have been attended by many instructors wishing to increase their knowledge and teaching abilities. In terms of faculty, more than 2,500 health instructors have been trained in these workshops. These instructors' skills have benefitted more than 26,000 health science students from the seven regional public health universities in Ethiopia.

This is a notable achievement in itself, but what has happened is that the training curricula in these seven universities now are standardized through the EPHTI mechanisms. The materials are compatible with the resources available in Ethiopia, so professors and students can now move from one university to another and not have their education or work interrupted. We later decided to comply with the request from the Ethiopian government to help train 30,000 health extension workers with the materials and workshops developed through the EPHTI.

These are some of the results and progress made possible by the fact that health workers have been trained; university systems have been set up for education; and a close, intimate, and permanent relationship has been developed among the government of Ethiopia, the health ministry, the education ministry, and donors. What The Carter Center hopes to accomplish with the lessons learned from the EPHTI model of training health professionals in low resource environments is to make it as easy as possible for other areas with limited resources to adopt similar programs and methods in order to train the health professionals needed to service communities in need.

President Jimmy Carter
39th President of the United States of America
Founder, The Carter Center, Atlanta, Georgia

Acknowledgments

It has been an honor and a privilege to participate in the writing of this book. The Ethiopia Public Health Training Initiative (EPHTI) of The Carter Center provided the setting, vehicle, and spark that allowed the teaching learning strategies presented herein to grow and flourish. The EPHTI would not be where it is today without the initial architecture and development by Dr. Dennis Carlson. Dr. Carlson was with EPHTI in the beginning, and he continues to be a guiding light in its mission today. Other invaluable staff of the EPHTI include Mr. Aklilu Mulugeta, who was the first staff member to come onboard with the initiative in its early years and was instrumental in keeping the program running, as well as managing the development of the initiative's 228 health learning materials; Ms. Meseret Tsegaw, another founding staff member of the EPHTI, who played a key role in maintaining business and administrative functions in the Addis Ababa field office; Mr. Assefa Bulcha, who coordinated the drought response and accelerated health officer training programs and has been a stalwart administrator; and Dr. Hailu Yeneneh, the dedicated resident technical advisor of the EPHTI, who possesses a depth of knowledge, passion, and a steady voice that has been a key influence in the success of the program. His commitment to his country and the health and future of his fellow countrymen and -women is an inspiration to us all. Addis Ababa–based staff who were instrumental in ensuring the 13 national-level teaching learning workshops over the last decade were executed smoothly, as well as keeping the EPHTI office humming like a well-oiled machine, include Mr. Fekadu Tsige, Ms. Mahlet Tilahun, and Ms. Yemsrach Mulugeta. Every one of our Ethiopian colleagues has been a pleasure to work with, and we are humbled to count them as friends.

Joyce P. Murray
Anna Frances Z. Wenger
Elizabeth A. Downes
Shelly B. Terrazas

xix

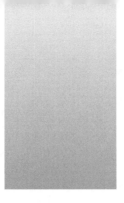

Introduction

This book is designed to engage teachers and students of the health sciences in the process of teaching and learning about the philosophy, methods, and strategies for the education of health care providers. It was written to be used in the preparation of teachers in preservice and in-service educational settings in low-resource countries and environments where material, technological, and electronic resources are often limited. Those who will find the book most helpful are teachers, experienced and new, who face the challenge of providing health science education in challenging settings. After more than a decade field-testing the methods and strategies described in this book in Ethiopia with a program at The Carter Center called the Public Health Training Initiative (PHTI), the model for teaching health professionals described herein is now applicable to most low-resource educational situations. The use of these teaching learning strategies within the PHTI program exemplify them as a successful mechanism that can be used in almost any low-resource setting. Featured in this book are active teaching learning strategies in which teachers and students work together to create learning situations that encourage critical thinking and creative problem solving.

Faculty and teachers in low-resource communities and countries face the issues of educating and preparing students with limited access to information for teaching and learning. *Low-resource environments* are those that have inadequate quantities and qualities of technological, electronic, and material resources, while at the same time the country (or county, school system, region, etc.) may have remarkable *human* resources. For an environment to be considered low resource, funding for resources for educational programs must be often lacking or limited.

BOOK STRUCTURE

The following 10 chapters, beginning with a description of teaching and learning, focus on the essential knowledge and skills needed by teachers who prepare health professionals. The first two chapters present the foundations for teaching learning, such as the definition of teaching and the theories and research supporting "active teaching learning strategies." Chapter three contains information on how the brain works, ways of knowing, and the theories behind learning strategies so a teacher can better understand his or her students. Chapters four and seven discuss instructional settings, while also addressing specific strategies for teaching, such as evidence-based methods, using teaching tools in the classroom, case studies, and service learning in conjunction with chapters five, six, and eight. Finally, chapters nine and ten of the book describe how an instructor would be a leader within the classroom, how to develop learning episodes, and how these tools worked in a thirteen-year project conducted in Ethiopia.

Topics presented include active teaching learning strategies, evidence-based teaching, learning theories, understanding the learner's learning style, incorporating culture, the dynamics of faculty–student relationships, and other methods and tools for preparing the health science student. Specific teaching strategies, such as problem-based learning, live patient scenarios, and simulation, are discussed. Emphasis within the chapters is on sources of information; the knowledge, skills, and attitudes needed for clinical practice; and the complex and important task of evaluation in both classroom and clinical settings. Another important aspect of being an effective teacher addressed is how to become a leader and role model for students.

At the end of many chapters are sections called *Learning Activities*, which are related to their respective sections in the chapter and titled accordingly. We have field-tested these learning activities for 10 years in Ethiopia as we conducted 2-week pedagogical skills workshops for health science instructors at the university level. These instructors, after participating in the pedagogical workshops that presented these learning activities, then conducted cascade workshops at their home institutions in which they replicated the learning activities. Most learning activities include a title, an overview, directions for student and teacher, and content sources that the teacher can use to conduct a teaching learning session and that the students can use when preparing for the session. The learning activities contain sources of information to adapt, plan, and implement the given learning activity. Also given within the learning activities are brief explanations referring the teacher to the strategies that guided the activity's development and relating to the specific topic under discussion.

Each learning activity is presented separately so that it can be copied directly from this book and used, or adapted, by teachers for their own educational settings. The learning activities can also serve as templates and guides for making similar learning activities that might fit better within the teaching learning context of the reader's educational setting.

HOW TO USE THIS BOOK

The organizational format of this book is meant to be flexible, and it can be used in multiple ways. Instructors with little to no background in education may use it as a reference guide to improve their knowledge and skills in teaching

---

Included Topics for Teachers

- Writing test questions
- Preparing lectures
- Utilization of problem-based learning
- Developing workshops on pedagogical skills
- Developing workshops on health service skills
- Knowing yourself as a teacher
- Faculty–student relationships
- Field trips
- Small group work
- Service learning
- Sources of information
- Simulation and role play
- Teaching in a classroom setting
- Teaching in a clinical setting
- Evaluation and assessment
- Critical thinking
- Developing a teaching learning episode

---

and learning. Topics can be reviewed in the order they are presented or used as references according to the reader's situational need. Topics include specific teaching skills, such as writing test questions, preparing a lecture, how to use problem-based learning, and developing workshops from 3 to 14 days in length that are focused on specific teaching and learning skills. The materials herein can also be used to structure, prepare, and conduct workshops for instructors on support skills as well as preparing health science students. Although 2-week workshop formats were used in the development of the material, the structure of the learning activities may also be adapted for shorter or more focused aspects of teaching and learning.

IMPROVING TEACHING PRACTICES THROUGH ACTIVE TEACHING LEARNING STRATEGIES

Although lecture has served as the major strategy and tool in teaching for many years, today the evidence shows that it is not in fact the most effective way to approach learning. New theories regarding how the brain works, and about the processing of information and learning, are providing evidence to support the theories of interactive teaching and learning. Research has uncovered information related to structuring learning experiences that enable students to use knowledge in new settings as well as information indicating that cultural and social norms influence learning and that new technologies will continue to impact effective teaching and learning. These new methods are called *active teaching learning strategies*, and they are discussed in chapters 4 through 7.

Another major deficit in teaching practices may be the absence of classroom resources such as culturally competent curricula, classroom teaching aids, computers, and anatomical models, for both teachers and students. Although the learning activities presented in this book are designed for low-resource environments that lack many of these items, the availability of such elements could be incorporated into a learning environment quite effectively.

Unfortunately, many faculty and instructors of health sciences receive little to no training as teachers. Often health professionals finish their educational programs and, because of situational needs, begin teaching immediately, with no formal training. The strategies in the chapters of this book were developed specifically in response to this scenario, which is seen frequently in environments with little resources for education. This book, which is meant to supplement formal educational training, was written for individuals who find themselves in a low-resource setting and must use their time and available resources as effectively as possible.

THE CRITICAL NEED FOR INCREASED HUMAN RESOURCES IN HEALTH

Dramatic global changes are occurring, yet low-resource countries still have inadequate, inappropriate, or unresponsive interventions to improve their health, education, social, and environmental situations. Health status has improved in some countries while deteriorating in others. Political changes in recent years in eastern Europe, the former Soviet Union, Africa, South America, and Asia led to expectations of a better life, including improved health care. Positive and negative changes in social development impact the lives of individuals and families in countries with low and high resources alike. Government services throughout the world vary in their abilities to meet the health care needs, including both availability and quality, of both rural and urban people.

The critical need for adequately prepared health care workers is clearly evident on a global scale. A 2006 World Health Organization report (Working together for health, The World Health Report) estimated a scarcity of health professionals that fell below the desired threshold of 80% coverage, which the WHO defines as a critical shortage. Thirty-six of the countries experiencing this health care human resource shortage are in sub-Saharan Africa. It is estimated that 2.4 million health professionals—an increase of almost 140% over current levels—would be needed to reach target levels for Africa.

Although the United States is a leader in basic health research, there are many parallels in health conditions in rural and poor urban areas in the U.S. and similar conditions in low resource countries. There are several factors in high- and low-resource countries that affect health conditions similarly. While poverty is more heavily concentrated in rural areas and poor urban areas, Bird, Hulme, Moore, and Shepherd (http://www.chronicpoverty.org/uploads/

publication_files/WP13_Bird_et_al.pdf), in their paper *Chronic Poverty and Remote Rural Areas* described remote rural areas worldwide as being most affected by poverty and poor health.

McGlaun and Cochran (2010) described barriers to health care access as a high number of uninsured persons, poverty, low educational level of women, lack of adequate transportation, and lack of health care providers. Recruitment and retention problems contribute to the lack of health care providers. Lack of education and living in remote rural areas tend to be correlated with poverty.

Health care worker shortages have created a global crisis situation. Further exploration of ways to increase the numbers of trained health professionals within diverse countries and communities, both with and without adequate resources, is desperately needed. The preparation of health workers requires organized, dedicated, and competent teachers to instruct and train the next generation of professionals for the delivery of quality care so that this urgent global health care need can be addressed.

PUTTING TEACHING LEARNING STRATEGIES TO WORK

In the 1990s, The Carter Center (a nongovernmental organization created by former U.S. President Jimmy Carter and based in Atlanta, Georgia) was asked by the Ethiopian government to help them address the lack of health professionals to meet the country's health care needs. The Carter Center's Public Health Training Initiative (PHTI) was conceived as one approach to, or model of, successful cooperation among a country's stakeholders in health (Ministry of Education; Ministry of Health; public universities; health bureaus; and funding sources, such as the U.S. Agency for International Development) to address the severe shortage of health professionals. One major component of the PHTI model is the preparation of university faculty to adequately teach their health science students. Without well-prepared teachers, increasing the numbers of quality health professionals will not be possible.

The PHTI in Ethiopia is described in detail in chapter 10 as an example of this book's strategies and methods in action. It was this program and teaching model, developed and conducted in a low-resource educational environment, that allowed us to field-test the teaching learning strategies and methods described. Although the teaching learning methods used in the PHTI project and detailed in this book were developed and used on a national scale, they can be effectively used in any environment and by any teacher faced with limited resources.

REFERENCES

Bird, K., Hulme, D., Moore, K., & Shepherd, A. Chronic poverty and remote rural areas (CPRC Working Paper No. 13). Retrieved from http://www.chronicpoverty.org/uploads/publication_files/WP13_Bird_et_al.pdf

McGlaun, J., & Cochran, C. (2010). *Rural Assistance Center: Women's frequently asked questions.* Retrieved from http://raconline.org/info_guides/public_health/womenshealthfaq.php

World Health Organization. (2006). *The World Health Report 2006: Working together for health.* Retrieved from http://www.who.int/whr/2006/whr06_en.pdf

1

What Is Teaching? What Is Learning? What Is Active Teaching Learning?

Multiple approaches to teaching and learning exist in today's learning environments. In the past, teaching consisted mostly of lectures and testing. Understanding the shift to active teaching and learning in education requires that one understand what it means to teach and learn. In fact, current research demonstrates that active teaching learning approaches are more effective than traditional approaches in the process of teaching learning. We begin this chapter by presenting a conceptual framework that shows the major concepts of an active teaching learning model (National Research Council, 2000).

A FRAMEWORK FOR ACTIVE TEACHING LEARNING

Active teaching learning refers to the interactive activities among learners, teachers, and other persons who may be involved in the process of teaching and learning in ways that promote critical thinking, creativity, and problem solving (Smith, 1990). The term *active teaching learning* is often used because teaching and learning interact and influence each other, often simultaneously. For many years, models of and approaches to teaching focused on lecture, testing, recitation, and written papers. Lecture has been, and often still is, the teaching strategy used most often in formal educational settings: Teachers talk, and students listen. In contrast to this historical method, recent research conducted by the U.S. National Research Council (2000) supports the science of how to link research findings regarding efficient learning to actual practices in classrooms.

Health science instructors come to the role of teacher with preexisting knowledge, beliefs, and experiences that influence how they teach and learn. Often, their preexisting perceptions consist of incomplete knowledge, false beliefs, and a naïve understanding of concepts related to teaching and learning (Graffam, 2007; Kaufman, 2003). These false beliefs and incomplete conceptual understanding of what it means to be a teacher must be clarified and corrected to help students rethink the role of the teacher and understand how people learn. Emphasis should be placed on understanding and doing, as opposed to rote memorization (National Research Council, 2000).

In many settings, at all levels of education, there are inadequate numbers of prepared, effective teachers, and teaching materials and technology are scarce. Most often, preparation of health professionals as teachers and educators is minimal at best. New graduates of health professional programs become teachers with only a scant background in education and no experience in teaching and learning. Health officers, advanced practice nurses, medical laboratory technicians, and environmental technicians are nonphysician health care providers who help fill the gaps in health care workers and teachers in local, rural, and regional areas in low-resource areas (Vanderschmidt et al., 1979). Teacher preparation is not part of the educational program in many health educational settings, yet many health professional graduates become teachers or preceptors almost immediately after graduation.

The goal of this book is to provide an active teaching learning model for preparing professionals from different health disciplines to become teachers. Theories supporting active teaching learning strategies are covered in depth in chapter 2. This book is structured around a framework, the Teaching Learning Framework, that supports active teaching learning strategies in multiple settings. The Teaching Learning Framework has six major categories, along with corresponding teaching strategies and activities to support each category (see Figure 1.1):

1. Philosophical Bases for Teaching and Learning
2. Teaching and Learning Context
3. Cultural Context
4. Teaching and Learning Setting
5. Personal Motivations and Goals
6. Teaching Learning Approaches

Each category, discussed in more detail later in this chapter, includes selected active teaching learning strategies. Figure 1.1 depicts how these six categories of the active teaching learning framework come together to describe what it is to teach. The figure pictorially demonstrates how teaching learning approaches, which are at the hub of the diagram, relate to all five surrounding categories. Throughout the book, we describe teaching learning approaches, usually referred to as *active teaching learning strategies*, as they apply to the topic under discussion.

Philosophical Bases for Teaching and Learning

Multiple definitions of *teaching*, *learning*, *training*, and *education* exist in the literature, and the terms are often used interchangeably, with little differentiation in the meanings of each. An understanding of the meaning of and differences between these terms is important, because teachers consider all of these concepts as they

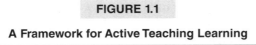

A Framework for Active Teaching Learning

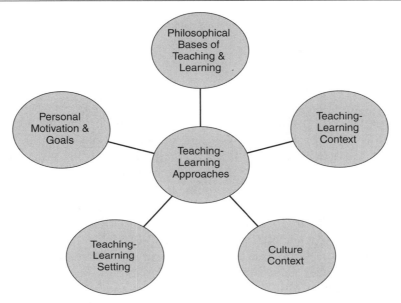

make decisions about approaches they will use to accomplish the identified learning outcomes. The effectiveness of one's teaching and evaluation is closely tied to the teaching strategies chosen to accomplish the outcomes and goals, which are determined before one begins to teach. Differentiation of the terms *teaching*, *learning*, *training*, and *education* helps to clarify ideas and concepts related to teaching and learning. Understanding the meanings of these terms also can help one understand how teachers create learning experiences; select testing strategies; and identify desired levels of learning as related to goals, objectives, and outcomes.

What is Teaching?

Each person's experiences and beliefs about teaching influence how he or she evolves into a teacher. *Teaching* is generally defined as telling or explaining ideas to others; however, the term can also mean that, through teaching, a person has influenced the life of another person in some meaningful way. Expanded definitions of *teaching* also include the acts of identifying a student's strengths and weaknesses and of helping a student develop his or her full potential in the subject of concern. The education of health professionals focuses on preparing a competent, safe, and caring practitioner dedicated to providing health care to diverse populations in many different settings. Educating health professionals is not about creating a simplistic, ritualistic practitioner. Because multiple definitions of teaching exist, and because teaching health professionals requires the combination of most of these definitions, the word *teaching* as used in this book refers to the act of influencing students—through teaching strategies, teacher–student interactions, selection of content, and methods of evaluation—to become well-rounded, competent health care practitioners who are prepared to practice in a multitude of settings.

What is Skillful Teaching?

Even the best prepared, most experienced teacher will face unpredictable and unanticipated situations. The experience of being a teacher will contain failures, ambiguity, joys, and frustrations; however, the most important focus for the teacher is the students' learning experiences and personal survival. Brookfield (1990) described teaching as an unpredictable and complex endeavor that is uncertain at times. He equated it to white water rafting, with periods of apparent calm interspersed with sudden, frenetic turbulence. Skillful teaching focuses on survival and being able to reduce negative experiences that lead to burnout, exhaustion, and the feeling that one is a failure. Brookfield advised educators to "be wary of the perfect teacher syndrome" (pp. 7–8). Indicators of a good teacher include the readiness to take risks, being realistic, and developing insights into who one is as a teacher. Developing a personal vision of who you are as teacher based on your instincts, intuitions, and insights that you gain over time will serve as a guide for your teaching career.

Definitions of teaching must be broad enough to include what skillful teaching is. In other words, does the teaching lead to students' success in their roles as health care workers in the environments in which they will practice? Sharing definitions and beliefs about teaching and learning leads to an understanding of teacher and student roles in the learning process.

What is Learning?

For our purposes, *learning* is defined as the act, process, or experience of gaining knowledge or skills in multiple ways. Two major models have influenced teaching and learning. The first, called the *behaviorist model* of learning, defines learning as a change in behavior and the acquisition of new knowledge or skills through study (DeYoung, 2003; Ironside, 2001). The behaviorist model has been widely known for its emphasis on behaviors: being able to explain what one has learned; pass the test; perform the skill; and, ultimately, to pass the course or receive the certificate. B. F. Skinner, an American psychologist known for his impact on education in the 1950s and 1960s, developed the behaviorist model as a means of focusing on behavioral objectives, objective test questions, and the student's ability to implement prescribed behaviors. Long the dominant paradigm in education, the behaviorist model has recently been contrasted with the second major model: the *human science model*, which is enjoying a growing influence on educational settings and is supported by the expanding use of technology.

The human science model of learning is a relatively new way of thinking among educators and scientists. As teachers, our philosophical beliefs about learning and our educational experiences are often reflected in our choice of teaching strategies and approaches that support our definitions of teaching and learning. Thomas Kuhn (1962), in his most renowned book, *The Structure of Scientific Revolution*, argued that science is not a steady, cumulative acquisition of knowledge, but rather a series of scientific developments following the scientific rules and regulations of the day as punctuated by intellectual explosions stimulated by new or different ways of thinking, which Kuhn called *scientific revolutions*. The shift from the behaviorist model to the human science model led to a revolution in both science and education. When a model that has been effective in making sense of phenomena in a given discipline at a particular time yields to another model, this is called a *paradigm shift*. The shift from the behaviorist model to the human science model has led to significant changes in health and education.

Table 1.1 illustrates and compares the behaviorist model and the human science model. Each model contributes to teaching and learning, but with emphasis on different strengths and differences.

TABLE 1.1
BEHAVIORIST MODEL VERSUS HUMAN SCIENCE MODEL

Behaviorist model[a]	Human science model[b]
1. Break down information and skills into small pieces.	1. Importance is placed on being in control of one's learning.
2. Check students' work regularly and provide feedback.	2. Students should be able to recognize what they know and do not know.
3. Teach out of context on the basis of the belief that students learn better when they are out of the context in which the learned material will be used.	3. Students recognize how they understand information.
4. Instruction is teacher centered; teaching strategies include lectures, tutorials, drills, and other teacher-controlled activities.	4. Students recognize how they have the ability to determine someone else's meaning and how one seeks evidence that supports his or her learning.
5. Learning is passive.	5. Learning is active.
6. Students must learn the correct response.	6. Students explore responses and make choices.
7. Knowledge is defined as remembering information.	7. Knowledge is defined as acquiring new information.
8. Understanding is defined as seeing existing patterns.	8. Students search for and create new patterns.
9. Applications require transfer of training, which requires one to see common elements among problems.	9. Students direct their own learning.
10. Teachers must direct the learning process.	10. Understanding is defined as creating new patterns.

[a] Adapted from: http://msucares.com/health/health/appa1.htm.
[b] Adapted from: http://viking.coe.uh.edu/~ichen/ebook/et-it/behavior.htm.

What is Training?

The term *training* generally refers to the acquisition of knowledge and skills (or competencies), developed through the teaching of vocational or practical skills. The words *training* and *education* are often used interchangeably, as though they mean the same thing, but it is important that teachers recognize their differences and that this recognition affects their choice of teaching strategies. Teachers often choose the behavioral model to help students prepare for specific tasks and roles supported by specific information (DeYoung, 2003; Ironside, 2001; Kaufman, 2003). Teaching skills to health workers generally includes training in which skills are matched to environments where graduates will work (see chap. 7, this volume). Skills training is essential to health professionals, but it is not sufficient. Understanding the principles and rationale behind skills, along with performance of those skills, is essential to preparing a safe practitioner.

What is Education?

Education, according to the human science model, builds a knowledge and theoretical base that can be transferred and used in other areas to continue growing and learning (Huitt, 2009). In health care, education focuses on personal development as well as training in the necessary skills and procedures with which health professionals must be familiar. In educating health professionals, teachers should encourage their students to pursue continued personal development and personal growth so that they can become competent professionals who can improve the delivery of health care to diverse populations. Education is essential to innovation and improvement. Incorporation of changes, new methods, and approaches are essential to providing safe, quality health care within the current health care system.

The Teaching Learning Context in Low-Resource Countries

The teaching learning context influences the work of students and teachers. The preparation of health professionals occurs in multiple settings, including classrooms, clinical settings, communities, and homes. The context in which teaching and learning take place influences those experiences as well as students' and teachers' ability to transfer that learning to other settings. Selection of teaching strategies and methods also is influenced by the context in which one works. Certainly, low-resource countries face many challenges in providing education to health professionals. Adequately prepared teachers and the availability of teaching resources, computers, and other technology are not readily available in low-resource countries. Also, health care systems in these countries often are not adequately equipped with the supplies, medications, and aides needed for teaching and providing care.

Although teaching in low-resource countries can be challenging and difficult, preparing teachers well in such countries can improve the quality of teaching and education, if only by strengthening the teachers' knowledge and skills.

Of course, effective teachers assume responsibility for identifying the content, strategies, and expected outcomes for what the students gain through engaged learning. Active teaching learning strategies engage the students in producing work while gradually turning over the learning process to students.

Cultural Context: Influence of Values, Beliefs, and Past Educational Experiences

Early basic education programs often provide the mindset for learning in later educational experiences. Personal learning styles based on initial educational experiences are often considered the only way to approach learning. This influence of prior experiences has been exemplified in stories from health professionals from various environments when they have been asked to share positive and negative experiences from their educational history (Wenger, 2008). Self-reflection yields stories that portray negative and positive experiences that shape who one is as a practicing health professional or teacher. The sharing of personal view–shaping stories with colleagues creates an open, supportive environment for new learning experiences. Examining the positive and negative aspects of personal influence also leads to a list of positive and negative teaching behaviors that illustrate the values and beliefs of who one is as teacher. Knowing one's self as a teacher influences the teacher–student relationships that are developed in the teaching learning process.

Understanding students' beliefs, values, and experiences helps teachers be more effective. A common language allows for easier communication between teacher and student. Also, understanding the culture, religious beliefs, roles of males and females, communication patterns, and other cultural traditions of the groups assists the teacher in creating a positive environment with a diverse group of learners. Please refer to Chapter 3 for more discussion on culture and learning.

Teaching and Learning Settings

The preparation of health care workers requires a variety of different settings that support active teaching learning strategies. Health educator preparation focuses on learning in classrooms; clinical settings, such as health centers and hospitals; homes; and other, nontraditional settings. Understanding how these environments influence the teaching learning process is necessary as well, because it enables the teacher to prepare experiences from which students can learn.

Teaching in the Classroom

Teaching in a classroom setting is challenging. It requires that teachers be adequately prepared so they can develop lectures, manage small and large groups, evaluate and assess students' learning, and use active teaching learning strategies. Although students often prefer the lecture format over participating in small group work or making presentations, teachers should keep in mind that student engagement necessitates a variety of teaching strategies. Topics related to classroom teaching are covered throughout this book. Skills that are needed for classroom teaching include an understanding of how students learn and come to know things. Understanding learning theories, ways of knowing, learning styles, how to write behavioral objectives and outcomes, writing test questions, plan and conduct a lecture, and understand and conduct student evaluation and assessment are all essential skills for classroom teachers.

Personal Motivation and Goals

Given that the greatest threat to world health is the shortage of health professionals, one of the most critical issues in the planning and improvement of better health care delivery is the training and education of health professionals who become teachers for their profession. Students entering health professional educational programs or learning programs to become health workers have expectations and goals, and they bring with them past educational experiences and an anticipation of learning new knowledge and skills that will make them competent practitioners and teachers. Meeting this expectation requires the teacher to understand learners' personal and group goals; clarify definitions related to teaching, learning, training, and education; and understand students' perceptions of effective teachers.

EVIDENCE-BASED TEACHING AND LEARNING

Many definitions of *evidence-based teaching and learning* exist, ranging from research-based information to expert practitioner opinions and theory-based information. The most commonly quoted definition of evidence-based teaching describes the use of current best practices and evidence to make decisions about the most effective teaching methods, which will result in increased learning for students and thus (theoretically) the best care of patients (Yannacci, Roberts, & Ganju, 2006). This definition provides insight into the essential components of *evidence-based practice*, a term that describes a process used in making safe, appropriate, and maximally effective decisions that are based on current research, clinical knowledge, and successful experiences. Because evidence-based practice is a process, decisions can and will change on the basis of the current available research, knowledge, and experiences. Although the evidence-based process varies in its descriptions (of how it works), common steps in teaching do exist. The following are some examples of these steps:

- Review and study the teaching learning environment, the situation, available readings, educational level of students,[1] information from the environment, and the issues arising out of an existing problem or problems.
- Identify and describe the issues/problems.

---

[1]Educational student level refers to whether a student is a beginner or more advanced in their program of study (i.e., first year or final year students). Expectations of students just beginning a program will be different than that of students who have more experience or education, and the evidence-based teaching strategies employed should take these various educational and experience levels into consideration.

- Construct questions that need to be answered.
- Review and evaluate the related literature and other sources of information and data related to the issue/problem. These sources should include current research; experts; practitioners; reputable Web sites; and information obtained in quality workshops, training, and courses.
- Return to the teaching situation with the information and evidence needed to implement successful teaching and learning.
- Monitor and evaluate to determine the effectiveness of the evidence in resolving and/or improving the situation.

Evidence-based teaching and learning practices are based on adult learning theories and, as the name implies, are supported by empirical evidence. Many reviews of adult learning theories have determined the knowledge and skills that focus on how adult learners learn (Yannacci, Roberts, & Ganju, 2006). The following three common principles of learning have been described:

1. Learners must be engaged by understanding the value and benefits of their learning.
2. Outcomes and goals are clearly defined.
3. Teachers should use evidence-based teaching principles to facilitate learning.

For many years, learning was based on psychological models that focused on individual tasks and the behavior changes that were necessary to accomplish those tasks (DeYoung, 2003; Kaufman, 2003). As discussed earlier, an alternative paradigm, the human science model, was presented. This model demonstrated that learning is specifically grounded in interactions between the learner and his or her social context, which helps to facilitate and reinforce the learning process (Kuhn, 1984). Active teaching learning strategies require involvement between teacher and students. Understanding who one is as teacher allows one to fulfill the role of teacher and supports the development of positive faculty–student relationships, facilitating the learning and growth of both teacher and student (Yannacci, Roberts, & Ganju, 2006).

What Is Evidence-Based Teaching/Education?

Evidence-based teaching is often described as the use of the most effective teaching strategies to accomplish desired outcomes for students/learners. Students learn more when evidence-based teaching methods are used than when traditional teaching methods (e.g., a lecture format) are used. Some professionals believe that evidence-based teaching and learning will be based on the best science, science that has been rigorously analyzed and has led to positive outcomes in regard to student learning. In fact, research shows that teaching strategies that require student participation result in increased student learning and retention of the learned material (National Research Council, 2000, pp. 3–6). Evidence-based education operates on two levels: (a) through the use of existing evidence from worldwide research and related subjects and (b) by establishing sound evidence where existing evidence is lacking or questionable.

Today the educational and health disciplines are exploring the processes of teaching and learning in conjunction with how the brain works. Evidence-based practices and teaching approaches are being implemented in educational settings worldwide with positive results. A basic approach to implementing evidence-based teaching practices involves the following steps for a teacher to undertake:

- Be able to pose the questions to be answered.
- Systemically and comprehensively search for evidence.
- Read and critique evidence according to professional and scientific standards.
- Organize and determine the levels of evidence. Randomized clinical trials are often seen as the gold standard in regard to evidence; however, sometimes practical wisdom, context sensitivity, and culture pervade medical and educational practices.
- Determine the evidence's relevance to educational needs and environmental conditions.
- Clearly describe the educational outcomes desired. Evidence is frequently defined as "what works."
- Evaluate and analyze the educational activity or health intervention.

Low-resource countries face challenges in obtaining research resources and often must depend on colleagues from other countries, experts, and other sources to access evidence-based information. Other sources of information include experts in the field; universities; the Internet; and research journals, where available. Last, but not least, consider the patient and the family as you consider the use of the evidence.

WHO AM I AS TEACHER?

Becoming a teacher is a journey of growth through personal experiences that leads one to determine who one is or wants to be as an educator. Depending on their educational experiences, beginning teachers often choose to emulate the style of one of their own favorite instructors. New teachers also purposefully avoid methods from past mentors and teachers with whom they did not connect.

As a teacher or educator, one brings into the classroom and other learning environments all of one's educational experiences, positive and negative, that shape who one is as a professional. Students often share stories about their positive and negative experiences with teachers and the impact of their connections with teachers on their overall learning. One's beliefs about oneself and others impact one's instructor–student relationships. Examining your own personal experiences and beliefs about personal and professional relationships helps you as a teacher focus on who you want to be as an educator. Experienced teachers often share stories that focus on how they have become the teachers they are today. Continuous growth and development help a teacher progress through the stages of development that come with experience.

LEARNING ACTIVITY 1.1

**CLARIFYING DEFINITIONS: TALKING THE SAME LANGUAGE
AND CHARACTERISTICS OF AN EFFECTIVE TEACHER**

PART I

The purpose of this learning activity is to clarify ideas and concepts related to teaching and learning. It is important that we share and understand the meanings and use of terms related to teaching and learning, that is, that we talk the same language. Sharing experiences and stories enriches our understanding of positive and negative episodes in our lives.

This is a guide to assist a group in a successful discussion of effective teaching. The outcome of this activity is that students will be able to discuss concepts that will serve as a beginning conceptual structure or mental model for teachers and educators.

Instruct students to read the lyrics to "Flowers are Red," a song written and sung by Harry Chapin that illustrates the impact teaching strategies have on students' learning. The song tells the story of a little boy on the first day of school. The boy was drawing pictures of flowers, using his imagination and a wide variety of colors to paint them. The teacher "corrects" him, telling him that he's using the "wrong" colors and that he should paint them red and green, "the way they always have been seen." The boy does not agree and continues to paint them from his imagination—until the teacher punishes the boy. The teacher stands him in a corner, until finally the little boy submits, repeating to the teacher her own words: "Flowers are red, and green leaves are green." The boy moves to a different school, and there he continues to routinely draw flowers in red and green, to the chagrin of his new teacher, who embraces individuality.

According to popular opinion, the idea for the song came to Chapin when his secretary told him about her son, who brought his report card home from school one day. The teacher had written a note in the card saying "Your son is marching to the beat of a different drummer, but don't worry, we will soon have him joining the parade by the end of the term." The quote was often used as an introduction to the song during live concerts. In the live concert versions, Chapin extended the song's ending to: "There still must be ways to have our children say. . ." before featuring the little boy's chorus again and bringing the song to a better conclusion.

The lyrics for the song can be found at *http://www.harrychapin.com/music/flowers.shtml* or *http://www.lyricsdepot.com/harry-chapin/flowers-are-red.html*.

The teaching strategies used in this activity are group discussion and Think–Pair–Share. Opportunities for students to be active in the learning process are inherent to group discussion. *Think–Pair–Share* is a collaborative learning strategy that has the following advantages: It can be used in very large classes, it encourages students to be reflective about the course content, it allows students to privately formulate their thoughts before sharing them with others, and it can foster higher order thinking skills (see *http://clte.asu.edu/active/usingtps.pdf*).

LEARNING ACTIVITY 1.2

CLARIFYING DEFINITIONS: TALKING THE SAME LANGUAGE AND CHARACTERISTICS OF AN EFFECTIVE TEACHER

PART II

After sharing and discussing the lyrics to the song "Flowers are Red," consider your definitions of *teaching*, *learning*, *training*, and *education*. Using a separate sheet of paper, write the definition of these four terms. Take a few minutes and do this.

As a group, discuss and share your answers to questions such as the following:

1. What is teaching?
2. What is learning?
3. What is training?
4. What is education?
5. What characteristics do you expect to see in an educated person?
6. What are the differences between training and education?
7. If learning does not take place, has teaching occurred?
8. Are your answers to these questions influenced by your beliefs, values, and past educational experiences? If so, how?

Following the discussion, put together a definition for each of these four terms: teaching, learning, training, and education. Continue to examine these terms as they relate to your work and to your development as a teacher.

LEARNING ACTIVITY 1.3
CLARIFYING DEFINITIONS: TALKING THE SAME LANGUAGE AND CHARACTERISTICS OF AN EFFECTIVE TEACHER

PART III

In this learning activity, share positive and negative educational experiences and discuss how they influence beliefs and values and who you are as learner and teacher. Reflection on positive and negative learning experiences provides an opportunity to share stories and to examine who you are or want to become as a teacher. This reflection will encourage you to consider and understand the importance of being in touch with and understanding your own humanity. It also will encourage the release of the human spirit in your teaching.

DIRECTIONS

A brief Think–Pair–Share exercise will be used in this assignment. Here is how it works:

1. **Think** about a positive and a negative encounter that you have had with a teacher at some time in your education experiences.
2. **Pair** with the person sitting next to you.
3. **Share** your positive and negative experiences together. Choose one negative and one positive response to share with the group.

Generate a list of positive and negative teacher characteristics.

Parker Palmer (1998), in his book *The Courage to Teach*, stated the following:

> Knowing my students and my subject depends heavily on self-knowledge. When I do not know myself, I cannot know who my students are. I will see them through a glass darkly, in the shadows of my unexamined life—and when I cannot see them clearly, I cannot teach them well. . . . I will know it only abstractly, from a distance, a congeries of concepts as far removed from the world as I am from personal truth. (p. 2)

He also stated that "good teaching cannot be reduced to technique; good teaching comes from identity and integrity" (p. 10).

Three important paths must be taken when one is preparing to become an educator: (a) intellectual, (b) emotional, and (c) spiritual. *Intellectual* refers to the way we think about teaching and learning, how people know and learn, the nature of our students and our subjects. Emotions are the feelings we have as we teach and learn. *Spiritual* refers to the heart's desire to be connected with the largeness of life—a longing that brings our teaching alive. (Palmer, 1998).

The table in Learning Activity 1.5 is designed to elicit and compare students' answers to the following questions:

- What is teaching?
- What is learning?
- What is training?
- What is education?
- How do our definitions and beliefs about each of these terms affect our approaches to teaching and learning?

Discussions of the answers to these questions will elicit rich exchanges of ideas and will help students identify and clarify each other's beliefs about teaching and learning and how these influence who one is as teacher and learner.

LEARNING ACTIVITY 1.5

**CLARIFYING DEFINITIONS: TALKING THE SAME LANGUAGE
AND CHARACTERISTICS OF AN EFFECTIVE TEACHER**

PART V

DEFINITIONS

Teaching	Learning	Training	Education

REFERENCES

Brookfield, S. D. (1990). *The skillful teacher*. San Francisco, CA: Jossey-Bass.

DeYoung, S. (2003). *Teaching strategies for nurse educators*. Upper Saddle River:, NJ: Prentice Hall.

Graffam, B. (2007). Active learning in medical education: Strategies for beginning implementation. *Medical Teacher, 29*, 38–42.

Huitt, W. (2009). *Humanism and open education*. Retrieved from http://www.edpsycinteractive.org/topics/affsys/humed.html

Ironside, P. M. (2001). Creating a research base for nursing education: An interpretive review of conventional, critical, feminist, postmodern, and phenomenological pedagogies. *Advances in Nursing Science 23*, 72–87.

Kaufman, D. (2003). ABC of learning and teaching in medicine: Applying educational theory in practice. *British Medical Journal, 326*, 213–216.

Kuhn, T. (1962). *The structure of scientific revolution*. Chicago, IL: University of Chicago Press.

Kuhn, T. (1984). *The structure of the scientific revolution*. Chicago: University of Chicago Press.

National Research Council. (2000). *How people learn: Brain, mind experience and school*. Washington, DC: National Academies Press.

Palmer, P. (1998). *The courage to teach*. San Francisco, CA: Jossey-Bass.

Smith, F. (1990). *To think*. New York, NY: Teachers College Press.

Vanderschmidt, L., Massey, J. A., Arias, J., Diong, T., Haddad, J., Noche, L. N., . . . Yepes, F. (1979). Competency-based training of health professions in seven developing countries. *American Journal of Public Health, 69*, 585–590.

Wenger, A. F. Z. (2008). *2008 Report on the 13th Teaching-Learning Workshop*. Atlanta, GA: The Carter Center.

Yannacci, J., Roberts, K., & Ganju, V. (2006). *Principles from adult learning theory, evidence-based teaching, and visual marketing: What are the implications for toolkit development?* Retrieved from http://ebp.networkofcare.org/uploads/Adult_Learning_Theory_2497281.pdf

2

Theories and Research Supporting
Active Teaching Learning Strategies

INTRODUCTION

Faculty in low-resource countries often become teachers with little or no preparation. In the absence of experience and knowledge provided by theories and research that support active teaching learning strategies, these faculty teach as they have been taught. Over the past 10 years, educational researchers have focused on teaching and learning from the perspectives of both teachers and learners. The Committee on Developments in the Science of Learning and Committee on Learning Research and Education, National Research Council (2000) conducted a study that linked research findings to actual teaching practices in the classroom and student outcomes. The purpose of this chapter is to explore how people learn and to examine learning theories and evidence-based research that support evidence-based teaching strategies, ways of knowing, and theories related to teaching and learning. Such a discussion helps frame the analysis of how and what we teach as well as identifies the goals and outcomes desired from teaching.

WAYS OF KNOWING

We now focus specifically on concepts related to the ways and means of building a knowledge base from which we educate teachers in the health sciences who will be training health care workers. Each health-related discipline builds its knowledge base through research, experiences, and skill development. We are required to look deeper into the roots of how choices are made regarding the nature of knowledge and how it affects the way we think, teach, and learn. Carper (1978) wrote a landmark article for the discipline of nursing about patterns of knowing. She identified four patterns that set the stage for how a health-related discipline places emphasis and value on particular types of knowledge, thus influencing how practitioners of that discipline provide health care services: (a) empirical knowledge, (b) personal knowledge, (c) moral knowledge, and (d) aesthetics. Phrased more specifically, the sources of knowledge that a health-related discipline favors influence the content that teachers in that specific discipline choose to focus on with their students. We discuss Carper's four patterns of knowing in more detail later in this chapter.

Knowledge Development

In order to understand how students learn, it is important to clarify various ways of knowing in the teaching learning process. In this respect, it is important to examine, if only briefly, the contemporary context of knowledge development in the health sciences. In 1977, Larry Laudun, a philosopher of science, claimed that the purpose of science was to solve problems—real live problems often posed by ordinary people in communities. He proposed that a theory should be judged by its effectiveness in solving problems rather than by its ability to confirm or disprove a scientific hypothesis. Until this time, most researchers, especially those in the natural sciences, had viewed empirical positivism as the major scientific paradigm from which to research cause–effect relationships.

Empirical positivism is a philosophy of science with this central tenet: Knowledge is based on sense experience with positive verification. In the positivist paradigm, the goal of research is to claim, or approach as closely as possible, unicausal relationships; that is, one causative agent relates to one perceived effect. For example, note the relationship between the tubercle bacillus (cause) and tuberculosis (effect); the former causes the latter. However, when dealing with issues in the natural world rather than in a laboratory, especially when problems relate to human beings, controlling for all potential causes and effects becomes an insurmountable task, thus giving rise to scientific studies whose methods allow for multicausal relationships.

In this respect, Laudun and others (Laudun, 1977; Polanyi, 1969) argued that knowledge is multifaceted and that professionals in the human sciences should embrace ways of knowing somewhat broader than those made available through empirical positivism (i.e., searching for scientific proofs using only empirical methods). This movement opened the way for science to include important nonempirical and nonscientific ways of knowing.

Patterns of Knowing

In her seminal work on patterns of knowing in nursing, Carper (1978) reported that "It is the general conception of any field of inquiry that ultimately determines the kind of knowledge the field aims to develop as well as the manner in which that knowledge is to be organized, tested and applied" (p. 13). Although Carper developed her thesis on patterns of knowing on the basis of "an analysis of the conceptual and syntactical structure of nursing knowledge" (p. 13), the four patterns of knowing that she identified apply equally well to all health-related disciplines.

We now provide a fuller description of the four patterns of knowing that Carper (1978) proposed. The first pattern, *empirical knowledge*, refers to what is generally called "science." Each health-related discipline conducts its own research in domains of inquiry specific to its field of practice while at the same time participating in the development of scientific knowledge in collaboration with other health disciplines. In addition, each health-related discipline uses scientific knowledge from the natural and social sciences.

The second pattern, *personal knowledge,* refers to knowing and understanding the self in relation to the other. Buber (1970) called this process the *I–Thou encounter*. This way of knowing is actualized through an interpersonal relationship. According to Carper (1978), the relationship is one of reciprocity, not only for the other person but also for oneself. Personal knowing takes place when the knowing and understanding of the self extend to other selves as well as to one's own self. In the health-related disciplines, personal knowing is essential because of the constant need for interpersonal communication on many levels. Carper suggested that personal knowing is often the most problematic, "the most difficult to master and to teach" (p. 18). Regardless of the setting, all health care workers need to become aware of the growing evidence indicating that the quality of interpersonal contacts influences health promotion and disease prevention efforts.

The third pattern of knowing is called *aesthetics,* or *perception knowledge.* Carper (1978) chose to call it *aesthetics* in the sense that health-related disciplines generally recognize that there is an art to professions such as nursing, medicine, medical laboratory technology, and environmental technology. What constitutes aesthetic knowledge may vary among health-related disciplines, yet all disciplines can acknowledge that *aesthetic expression*—that perceptive process of gathering together bits and pieces of a situation into an experienced whole for the purpose of seeing what is there—characterizes it as aesthetic or perception knowledge. For example, "The experience of helping must be perceived and designed as an integral component of its desired result rather than conceived separately as an independent action imposed on an independent subject" (Carper, 1978, p. 17).

All health care workers use aesthetic patterns of knowing, although few would recognize the theoretical underpinnings that give rise to these important actions. Also, teachers often unknowingly expect perceptive qualities to be present in their students while at the same time offering little guidance for the development and use of perception or aesthetic knowledge. For example, empathy—the capacity for participating indirectly or vicariously in another person's feelings—is a mode of an aesthetic pattern of knowing. The more skilled a health care worker becomes in perceiving the lives of other people, the greater will be his or her ability to understand various modes of perceiving reality (Carper, 1978). This larger repertoire of choices in designing assistive and therapeutic options also increases the complexity of the individual's decision-making process. Such increased complexity can be aided by additional aesthetic and perceptive ways of knowing, such as creativity, imagination, inventiveness, visualization, discernment, and intuition.

The fourth and final pattern of knowing involves *moral knowledge*. Ethics is increasingly recognized as an essential component of educational programs and practice settings for all health workers. The ethical component of knowing focuses on matters of obligation—what ought to be done, what was omitted, and what was done that ought not to have been done. However, knowing the ethical rules is not enough; moral knowledge also includes voluntary action that is subject to an analysis of right and wrong.

Because there are differences among cultures in terms of specific judgments of right and wrong, the contextual setting is important. Indeed, understanding the contextual setting is vital to providing appropriate and effective health care. At the same time, the contextual setting enters into the determination of moral understanding and ethical rules, which may complicate situations in relation to universally accepted ethical standards within specific health-related disciplines. In brief, health care workers must be aware of the moral and ethical codes of the cultural context within which they are practicing, in addition to the universally accepted code of ethics and moral knowledge of their own discipline. Munhall and Oiler (1986) summarized the requirements of this domain as understanding the following four things: (a) ethical theories, (b) conditions of society, (c) conflicts between different value systems, and (d) ethical principles.

Although these patterns of knowing may seem like discrete, separate categories, they are not; they are interdependent and not exclusive of one other. The challenge for the teacher is to examine all curricular sections and ask the following question: "Have I included opportunities to introduce students to all relevant ways of knowing, so that they can understand the interdependence of empirical knowledge, aesthetic knowledge, personal/interpersonal knowledge, and moral/ethical knowledge?"

Participatory Education

Before leaving this discussion on ways of thinking, it is important that we mention Brazilian educationalist Paulo Freire, whom some consider the most influential thinker in education of the late 20th century. Freire (1972, 1995) left a significant mark on thinking about progressive practice (Smith, 1997/2002). He focused on informal education, with an emphasis on dialogue with and concern for the oppressed. He drew on and wove together a number of strands of thinking about educational practices and liberation. Aspects of his work that are worth noting as essential elements that are applicable to both formal and informal education are listed in Exhibit 2.1. One can see that each of the essential elements listed in Exhibit 2.1 espouses participatory education. Freire viewed education as being a continuous interchange between teacher and student—or, as he called them, "educator and educatee"—in which both are teaching and learning.

Some of Freire's writing is quite dense, but it discusses many important components that have been proven to work in informal and formal education (Taylor, 1993). In fact, Freire's books have been used in many parts of the world,

EXHIBIT 2.1

Freire's Essential Elements of Education

- Dialogue that involves respect
- Praxis: action that is informal and linked to values
- Consciousness that has the power to transform reality
- Learning that is situated in the lived experience of the participants
- Transformation in which educators–educatees become educatees–educators

likely because he was able to weave together several strands of educational practice and liberation (Smith, 1997/2002). Smith (1997/2002) contended that Freire's (1972) *Pedagogy of the Oppressed* is currently one of the most often-quoted educational texts, especially in Latin America, Africa, and Asia. Two authors, Anne Hope from South Africa and Sally Timmel from the United States, have made Freire's educational ideas more accessible to the general public, especially in Africa, with their four volumes of *Training for Transformation* (Hope & Timmel, 1984, 1999). In these volumes, Hope and Timmel included line drawings of African scenes depicting aspects of the educational tenets discussed in text. Books 1, 2, and 3 are sold as a set and should be used as a combination reference of educational concepts and exercises based on Freire's educational works. Book 4 was published by Hope and Timmel in 1999 and extends Freire's ideas, but with development of topics such as environment, gender and development, racism, culture, and transforming governance.

At the end of this chapter we present Learning Activity 2.1, which further illustrates how teachers can engage students or workshop participants in using active teaching learning strategies related to ways of knowing. Please note the use of content mapping within this learning activity. Content mapping is a method for analyzing and organizing information in meaningful ways in order to visualize the relationships among the various types of content.

THEORIES OF ACTIVE TEACHING LEARNING STRATEGIES

Health professionals in many countries have expressed concern over the quality of health workers' professional education and the need to increase practitioner competency. Much has been written about the best way to teach and prepare an educated, competent practitioner. As researchers learn more about how the brain works, they have developed evidence-based teaching approaches and explored new educational strategies. But what, in fact, is evidence-based teaching and learning? How does it differ from the well-known behaviorist model, which is based on specific behaviors? How does it differ from the human science model? (See chapter 1 of this volume, for a discussion of the behaviorist model and the human science model.) What are the similarities and differences?

A variety of approaches have been used to support teaching and learning practices. Examples include tradition (i.e., "That's the way we have always done it"; "That is how I was taught"), authority, trial and error, personal experiences, and intuition. The field of neuroscience is now providing evidence for a variety of learning principles and theories. Laboratory research conducted by cognitive and developmental psychologists is providing evidence for many principles that support active teaching learning strategies. In addition, there is a growing recognition that teaching and learning take place in a variety of settings, with a particular set of cultural and social norms, with expectations that these settings influence teaching, learning, and the transfer of information.

What Is a Learning Theory? What Is a Model?

A *learning theory* is a general explanation or group of principles that explains and/or predicts facts, observations, or events (see http://www.learning-theories.com/definitions). Learning theories are generally considered valid foundations on which to base approaches to teaching and learning; however, a theory is not established beyond all doubt but is generally accepted as valid only after repeated successful usage and testing. A *model* is a theoretical construct or a picture that shows how the model works and leads to increased understanding of the construct at hand. Descriptions of four learning theory models—(a) constructivism, (b) Kolb's (1984) experiential learning, (c) situational learning, and (d) apprenticeships—are provided in the following sections.

Constructivism

Based on the earlier works of Dewey (1915) and Piaget (Boden, 1979), *constructivism* is a theory regarding how people think and learn. The underlying principle of constructivism is that individuals construct their understanding and knowledge of the world by experiencing events and reflecting on those experiences (Hein, 1996). This definition leads a teacher to a number of different teaching practices, with the goal that students will construct knowledge for themselves. New experiences must be reconciled with previous knowledge and experiences. This may lead one to change his or her beliefs and ways of doing things, or to discard new information. The learner is the creator of his or her own knowledge. Teachers must focus on the learner with the understanding that learners construct knowledge for themselves. Knowledge is not outside but must be constructed within, and by, the student in the process of learning.

Active teaching learning strategies used by teachers working within constructivist theory include questions, exploration, and accessing what one already knows. In general, constructivism includes using active teaching learning strategies and encouraging students to reflect on and assess how the activity is helping them to gain an understanding that helps them become expert learners. This view of constructivism is contextual, in that learners construct knowledge for themselves on the basis of the principles of learning, and it is an active process in which students use sensory input and motivation, both of which are essential for learning.

Kolb's Experiential Learning

We now turn to *experiential learning*, which can be characterized two ways: (a) It is learning in which students have the opportunity to acquire and apply knowledge, skills, attitudes, and feelings in an immediate, relevant setting, and (b) it is a direct encounter with a situation or phenomenon being studied. Thus, experiential learning involves a direct encounter with the phenomenon being studied or the task to be performed (Smith, 2001).

The learning cycle can begin at any one of four points: (a) concrete experiences, (b) observation and experience, (c) forming abstract concepts, and (d) testing in new situations. Kolb and Fry (1975) argued that the learning cycle can start at any point and works like a spiral. Five steps must be taken to fully realize Kolb's experiential learning model (Smith, 2001):

1. Carry out a particular action and observe the effects of the action in the situation.
2. Understand and describe the effects of the action in this particular situation so that it would be possible to anticipate and compare the reaction in other similar situations.
3. Repeat the action in a similar situation and compare the results.
4. Form abstract concepts that reflect the situation.
5. Continue to make comparisons in similar situations.

These steps help students make connections among situations, actions, and learning. The terms *experiencing, reflecting, conceptualizing*, and *experimenting* describe the process of experiential learning, which often is visualized as a spiral or wheel. Two characteristics are especially noteworthy: (a) the use of immediate experiences to test ideas and (b) the use of evaluations to change practices and ideas (Kolb, 1984).

Situational Learning

Situational learning includes many methods and approaches that focus on real life situations (Online Education, University of Adelaide, Australia, 2010). The environments in which students learn and function vary widely, just as students do. Today, students are looking for more active learning situations, including technology, where available. Contemporary educators should encourage the move from the standard lecture format to interactive teaching strategies that engage students in the learning process. Situational learning provides opportunities for educators and learners to analyze and synthesize; be creative; develop interpersonal skills; be a leader; use technology; and be aware of ethical, professional, and social issues. Technology has increased the possibilities of providing situational learning. Online materials such as case studies, group activities, and other strategies can support situational learning. Students can work individually or in groups on case studies; simulations; and interactions with patients, families, and small groups. Approaches such as these are engaging, interactive, and relevant to real life, and they provide opportunities for students to build the skills they will need when practicing in the field.

Certain skills can be obtained only through clinical practice. Students need opportunities to strengthen thinking skills such as analysis, synthesis, interpersonal understanding, teamwork and communication; also, to be competent in today's multicultural environments they need an awareness of social and cultural differences. Being able to work in situations that vary across disciplines is essential to providing safe, quality clinical care.

Apprenticeships

Apprenticeships are a bridge between the world of education and the world of work. They provide an opportunity for young people to train while in a job, obtain the necessary qualifications, and earn a wage. For employers, apprenticeships are a chance to recruit highly motivated staff and train them in the skills their business needs.

The aim of an apprenticeship is to boost skill levels in the workforce and help individuals become more productive, innovative, and competitive. Apprenticeships provide the opportunity for students to strengthen their skills and become more qualified and better prepared for the real world of work. It also allows for training in key skills such as information technology, teamwork, and effective communication. Most faculty will be able to assist students in locating information on how to seek and obtain apprenticeships in their professional area of health care.

Clinical practice apprenticeships serve as step between education and practice in the real world. Students benefit from practice within the educational programs, and being able to actually put their knowledge into practice helps strengthen their knowledge and skills as beginning practitioners.

LEARNING ACTIVITY 2.1
WAYS OF KNOWING

In this chapter we have discussed sources of information and the differences and similarities between information and knowledge. Each discipline works to build its knowledge base through research, experience, and skill development. The focus of this learning activity is on ways of knowing. This requires that you take a look deeper into the roots of how choices are made regarding the nature of knowledge and how it affects the ways people think, teach, and learn. Carper (1978) wrote a landmark article for the discipline of nursing about four patterns of knowing: (a) empirical knowledge, (b) personal knowledge, (c) moral knowledge, and (d) aesthetics. These four patterns apply equally well to any of the health science disciplines. The challenge and opportunity is for us, together, to make these and related concepts practical and relevant to the work of health professionals in whatever location we are living.

1. **Read Carper's article and the Patterns of Knowing worksheet provided in Learning Activity 2.1.**
   Use Learning Activity 2.1 to list one example of course content you teach that represents the pattern of knowing in that column. Do this for each of the four patterns of knowing.
2. **Read about Brazilian educationalist Paulo Freire's concepts about ways of knowing that are related to teaching and learning (see Smith [1997 and 2002]).** Think about the differences and similarities among knowledge learned from science, discipline-specific knowledge bases, traditional knowledge, and popular education of the people.

   Freire has been referred to as one of the most influential thinkers about teaching and learning in the late 20th century, especially because of his emphasis on dialogue with and concern for the oppressed. He was concerned with dialogue, working together, praxis, community capacity, social capital, conscientization, and experience of the participants.

   Question: Considering Freire's perspective, what are its implications for educating health professionals and enhancing the effectiveness of the community health centers in your part of the world?

Learning Activity 2.1   Ways of Knowing: Patterns of Knowing Worksheet (*Continued*)

In the spaces provided, give an example of course content in your discipline related to the type of knowledge in that column.

Empirical knowledge	Personal/ interpersonal knowledge	Aesthetic/perception knowledge	Ethics/moral knowledge
Emphasis is on the generation of theory and research that are systematic and controllable by factual evidence for the purpose of describing, explaining, and predicting phenomena of concern for the specific discipline. This knowledge is generally referred to as *science* and is assumed to form the major knowledge base in the health sciences. The next three patterns of knowing are now being recognized as essential components also.	Emphasis is on knowing the self and knowing other persons while striving toward authentic interpersonal communication and relationships. It is the most difficult to master and to teach within the health science disciplines. The therapeutic use of self strives always toward actualizing an authentic personal relationship between two or more persons.	Emphasis is on the ability to receive and express impressions. This calls for understanding intuition and feelings. An important mode of expression is *empathy*, the capacity for participating in or vicariously experiencing another person's feelings. The more skilled one becomes in perceiving the lives of others, the more knowledge one gains of alternate modes of understanding reality.	Emphasis is on matters of obligation, or what ought to be done. This domain requires an understanding of ethical theories, societal conditions, cultural values and beliefs, and ethical principles that may guide action. Moral choices need to be understood in terms of practical actions to be taken in specific concrete situations.

Note. For more information see Barbara Carper's article, "Fundamental Patterns of Knowing in Nursing," Advances of Nursing Science, 1(1), 1978, pp. 13–23.

In-Class Exercise	Using patterns of knowing to ascertain the sources of knowledge
	Active teaching learning exercise: content mapping
	Think about the content areas on some aspect of malaria that you would use when preparing a class session for senior-level students.
Subject	Content areas related to the prevention and control of malaria.
Question	What patterns of knowing might you use as you prepare to teach senior-level students?
Action Steps	1. Identify several content areas related to a class session on some aspect of the prevention and control of malaria.
	2. Write each content area on a separate Post-It note.
	3. Decide which pattern of knowing (Carper, 1978) best describes each content area.
	4. Attach each content area Post-It onto the appropriate pattern-of-knowing newsprint on the wall.

When all persons have put their content area Post-Its on the appropriate pattern-of-knowing paper on the wall, please note the following:

1. Do the outcomes cluster around any pattern of knowing?
2. If so, why might that have happened?
3. Which pattern of knowing received the most attention?
4. How might you become more aware of the sources of knowledge and patterns of knowing you use in your teaching?

Items needed for this exercise:

- 3 × 3-inch Post-It notes, or colored paper cut into 3-inch squares, and masking tape or Scotch tape
- Four large sheets of plain newspaper. At the top of each sheet, use a broad-tip felt-tip pen to write one pattern of knowing on each sheet. Attach the sheets to the wall with masking tape or Scotch tape. Allow space between each sheet so that the students can have space to stand while attaching their Post-It notes to the appropriate sheets of newsprint.

REFERENCES

Boden, M. A. (1979). *Piaget*. London, England: Fontana.

Buber, M. (1970). *I and thou* (W. Kauffman, Trans.). New York, NY: Charles Scribner's Sons.

Carper, B. A. (1978). Fundamental patterns of knowing in nursing. *Advances in Nursing Science, 1*, 13–23.

Committee on Developments in the Science of Learning and Committee on Learning Research and Education, National Research Council. (2000). *How People Learn; Brain, Mind, Experience, and School; Expanded Edition*, Washington, DC: National Academy Press.

Dewey, J. (1915). *The school and society*. Chicago, IL: University of Chicago Press.

Freire, P. (1972). *Pedagogy of the oppressed*. Harmondsworth, England: Penguin.

Freire, P. (1995). *Pedagogy of hope: Reliving pedagogy of the oppressed*. New York, NY: Continuum.

Hein, G. E. (1996). *Constructivist learning theory*. Retrieved from http://www.exploratorium.edu/ifi/resources/constructivistlearning.html

Hope, A., & Timmel, S. (1984). *Training for transformation: A handbook for workers* (Books 1, 2 and 3). Gweru, Zimbabwe: Mambo Press.

Hope, A., & Timmel, S. (1999). *Training for transformation: A handbook for community workers* (Book 4). London, England: ITDG Publishing.

Kolb, D. A., & Fry, R. (1975). Toward an applied theory of experiential learning. In C. Cooper (Ed.), *Theories of group process* (pp. 33–58). London, England: Wiley.

Kolb, D. A. (1984). *Experiential learning; Experience as a source of learning and development*. Englewood Cliffs, NJ: Prentice Hall.

Laudun, L. (1977). *Progress and its problems: Towards a theory of scientific growth*. London, England: Routledge & Kegan Paul.

Munhall, P. L., & Oiler, C. J. (1986). *Nursing research: A qualitative perspective*. Norwalk, CT: Appleton-Century-Crofts.

Online Education, University of Adelaide, Australia. (2010). *Situational learning*. Retrieved from http://www.adelaide.edu.au/situationallearning/sl/

Polanyi, M. (1969). *Knowing and being*. Chicago, IL: The University of Chicago Press.

Smith, M. K. (2001). David A. Kolb on experiential learning. In *The encyclopedia of informal education*. Retrieved from http://www.infed.org/biblio/b-explrn.htm

Smith, M. K. (2002). Paulo Freire and informal education. In *The encyclopedia of informal education*. Retrieved from http://www.infed.org/thinkers/et-freir.htm (Original work published 1997)

Taylor, P. (1993). *The texts of Paulo Freire*. Buckingham, England: Open University Press.

3

Understanding the Learner

Understanding the learner should be a prime concern of every teacher. Parker Palmer, in his book *The Courage to Teach* (1998), discussed the importance of creating community in the classroom: "The real threat to community in the classroom is not power and status differences between teachers and students but the lack of interdependence that those differences encourage" (p. 139). Palmer suggested that teachers and students are ideally interdependent, that is, they depend on one another in various ways. The question for us, then, is "In what ways are students and teachers interdependent?" It would be easy to create a list of ways that students are dependent on teachers; evaluations and grades would likely lead the list. It is more difficult, however, to think of the ways teachers are dependent on students. When interdependence is considered to be of prime importance in the teaching learning process, teachers will seek ways to promote a community of learning in which interdependence is expected: Teachers will be engaged in learning while they are teaching, and students will be engaged in teaching while they are learning. This kind of teaching learning atmosphere will direct the teacher's attention toward ways of understanding the cultural milieux, the diversity of the learning styles, and faculty–student relationships. All of these topics are covered in this chapter.

WESTERN AND NON-WESTERN CULTURES AND EDUCATION

During the current period of globalization, with its movement of students and teachers across national boundaries, one may wonder whether educational programs, cultures, and learning styles have become intermingled to the extent that former historical and geopolitical designations are no longer significant. Although labels such as *Western* and *non-Western* may be questioned because of the stereotypes associated with them, they are still relevant in relation to some cultural markers they bear. These markers will be discussed after a few remarks about the intended meaning of these terms, which clearly were developed by Westerners. Reagan (2005) asserted that

> The assumptions and stereotypes that need to be challenged are already present, and if our language reflects them then it may be useful to recognize the biases that are inherent in the language that we use. Thus, what begins as a false dichotomy can emerge as an effective way of challenging and reforming racist and ethnocentric assumption[s] and biases, both conceptually and linguistically. (p. 11)

In general, the terms *Western civilization* and *Western culture* refer to those that originated in Europe; some of them are still located in Europe, and others have spread to other parts of the world through migration and colonization. The term *Western cultures* refers to those in Europe, the Americas, and Australasia. Non-Western cultures usually include those in Africa, Asia, India, the Middle East, and sometimes Latin America and the Caribbean. These distinctions are made here for the sole purpose of calling attention to the cultural markers that often have a bearing on teaching learning situations, especially in regard to teachers or students whose formative years were spent in one part of the world and who then study or teach in another part of the world.

   Cultural markers are the specific values, beliefs, behavioral expectations, traditional customs, and patterns of thinking that characterize particular cultures and educational systems. Most Western cultures place a high value on individualism, human rights, problem solving, change, innovation, competition, and technology. By comparison, many non-Western cultures may be more likely to emphasize family and clan; community; honor of and respect for past traditions; collaboration; and the collected wisdom of elders, authority figures, and history. Teachers and students who teach or study in countries or communities where the educational systems and cultures differ from their own would do well to consider the impact of cultural similarities and differences and the way these similarities and differences may affect the ways they teach and learn. Imagine the cultural dissonance that might result when a teacher from the United States sets up a classroom exercise that is based on competition and requires intense verbal communication among students while he or she is teaching a health sciences course in East Africa, where other forms of interchange prevail. Achieving an understanding of the local educational system and cultural patterns and preferences is always recommended when students or faculty cross cultural boundaries.

CULTURE AND LEARNING

We turn now to some significant relationships between culture and learning. The first issue to consider deals with how a teacher understands his or her own culture and the various cultures that may be represented in his or her classroom, community, or clinical setting. The second issue addresses how teachers develop and practice cultural openness themselves and how they can encourage cultural openness among their students or workshop participants. Before we address these issues, let us offer some relevant definitions.

Concepts

Culture

The concept of culture can be defined in many ways, but within the context of the human sciences an anthropological meaning is most relevant. *Culture* refers to the sum total of the life ways of a group of people who share values, beliefs, and practices that are passed from generation to generation and that change over time (Leininger, 1991, Leininger & McFarland, 2006, Wenger, 1993). Culture is always an inherent part of life of all peoples in all countries, although it becomes more apparent when there are groups of people in close proximity whose life ways differ sharply. The term *life ways* refers to the shared patterns of daily life, customs, social systems, values, beliefs, and practices related to socially accepted gender roles; rituals; and *worldviews*, that is, the sense of self in relation to the universe. It is important to note that shared cultural life ways are patterned, learned, and passed from one generation to the next.

Culture has several other important features that relate to teaching and learning. Cultural life ways do change over time, with some changing more rapidly than others. In general, in regions where tradition and history are respected and honored, cultural changes may happen more slowly than in areas of the world that tend to orient more toward the future. Urban cultures, where technology and electronic innovations are more readily available, are more likely to change at a faster rate than rural cultures. In rural cultures, of course, technology can be minimal, and contact with persons outside the culture can be rare.

In Hall's (1976) *context-dependency model of communication*, high-context cultures gain meaning, or most meaning, through explicit expression within the culture, whereas low-context cultures gain meaning, or most meaning, implicitly, that is, within the transmitted message such as in verbal and written communication. For example, in a low-context culture like the United States, where people tend to be mobile and there is variability among many sub-cultures, written signs and instructions tend to be more frequent and elaborate. Whereas in low-context cultures, such as in rural communities in Africa, where people tend to be less mobile and share many life activities, a gesture or an abbreviated verbal communication may suffice, because much of the meaning is embedded within the context of past experiences. Readers should keep in mind that even in countries where the dominant culture is very low context (Hall, 1976; Wenger, 1991), such as in the United States, there can be many subcultures that are high context, such as ethno-religious cultures (e.g., the Old Order Amish, or immigrant communities whose members share language, life ways, and learning styles from cultures in their homelands). In high-context cultures, where people know each other over long periods of time, they learn to communicate more through shared understood meanings and inferences, along with body language (as in a knowing glance), than people in low-context cultures do. Because of less shared contextual meaning, effective communication in low-context cultures is more dependent on detailed messages and elaboration in verbal and written interactions. This brings us to our next concept: cultural boundaries.

Cultural Boundaries

Anytime you meet a person whose shared values, beliefs, and practices (life ways) are different than your own, you are encountering a *cultural boundary*. At this point, two things need to happen: You must (a) consider your own cultural self in order to understand one's personal contribution to the interaction and (b) consider how you will successfully relate to people whose culture is different than your own. Definitions of cultural boundaries vary according to disciplines, such as anthropology and business or finance, and according to the topic under discussion. For our purposes, the term *cultural boundaries* refers to the recognition of the differences and similarities between two or more cultures within a particular community, especially where teaching and learning contexts are concerned. In general, a boundary exists when insiders know they belong and outsiders know they do not.

Boundaries are not where things separate but where things join (Gunderson, 2004, p. 10). Learning to cross cultural boundaries is an essential part of a teacher's repertoire of knowledge, skills, and attitudes in relating to learners in classroom and health care settings. Viewing a cultural boundary as an opportunity rather than an obstacle should be an instructor's modus operandi when they encounter students, colleagues, or staff members from different cultures. Exhibit 3.1 lists the recommended requirements for crossing cultural boundaries. The following discussion on cultural openness can help prepare readers for crossing cultural boundaries effectively.

Cultural Openness

A commitment to cultural openness is essential for crossing cultural boundaries, whereby teachers and learners interact in the presence of cultural differences (Wenger, 1999). "Cultural openness refers to a life-long stance that

---

EXHIBIT 3.1

Requirements for Crossing Cultural Boundaries

- Cultural self-awareness
- Openness to learning from people whose cultures are different
- Knowledge about the cultures in the country, region, community, and place of work
- Knowledge about the cultures of one's colleagues and students
- Culture-crossing skills

promotes cultural self awareness and continuing development of transcultural skills" (Wenger, 1998, p. 164). Cultural openness has three essential components: (a) a lifelong commitment to the journey of becoming culturally open, (b) cultural self-awareness, and (c) continuing development of culture-crossing skills.

These three components will be discussed separately. First, a *lifelong commitment* requires one to look inward and to consider whether one wants to make a commitment to cultural openness, to taking a learner's stance in trying to understand the life ways of people who are different from the people of one's own culture. Here, personal commitment allows one to move forward, pointing one's actions toward mutual understanding of and respect for other cultures and ways of thinking and doing. Equally important is understanding that this commitment continues; it is a lifelong journey, and although it does not end, it will become more natural as time goes by. Of course, we all need to allow ourselves the freedom to fail when attempting cross-cultural teaching and learning opportunities—and failure will occur. Important here, though, is the context, the lifelong commitment to the journey that is "directed toward learning about cultural diversities while seeking common ground in cultural universalities" (Wenger, 1999, p. 10).

Cultural self-awareness is the second essential component of cultural openness. It, too, calls for one to look inward to gain increased cultural self-understanding. Cultural self-awareness is the linchpin of the cultural openness process, and it is hard work; however, the "Culture and Learning" exercise (Learning Activity 3.1) at the end of this chapter has two exercises designed to assist in the development of cultural self-awareness. In-Class Exercise 3.1 is called "Looking at Your Cultural Interface." The questions invite the individual to think about specific patterns of daily life, ways of thinking, health and illness behaviors, values and beliefs, and intra- and intercultural variations. For some people, one of the hardest parts of this exercise is to think of themselves as being part of a particular culture, because cultural differences have for them been a part of looking *outward* at other people who have different life ways. Cultural self-awareness addresses the need to look *inward* and at how a person presents him- or herself to others.

The third essential component of cultural openness is the continuous development of *culture-crossing*, or *transcultural skills*. Developing and using these skills continues throughout our lifetimes. The tendency toward ethnocentrism serves us well in that it helps the members of each cultural group love and understand their own culture best. Cultural identity is part of knowing who we are as compared with other groups of people, and it helps to shape our worldview, the way we see ourselves as part of the universe. Transcultural skills help teachers to better understand themselves and the learning styles of their students.

Culture and Learning Styles

Culture is intricately related to learning styles and learning preferences. Romanelli, Bird, and Ryan (2009) cited several authors (e.g., De Vita, 2001; Grasha, 1990) who have proposed that there are correlations between culture and learning styles. These correlations are "predicated on the concept that culture influences environmental perceptions which, in turn, to some degree determine the way information is processed and organized. The storage, processing, and assimilation methods, for information, contribute to how new knowledge is learned" (Romanelli et al., 1990, p. 3). For example, persons who lived most of their lives in cultures where literacy is emphasized tend to prefer written instructions and assignments, whereas persons who grew up in cultures with rich oral traditions tend to prefer oral discourse and they commit oral assignments and instructions to memory more readily.

The relationship between specific cultures and preferred learned styles has in recent years been questioned more frequently with the increase in globalization and the intra- and international movement of people. In Fierro's (1997) research article, "Is There a Difference in Learning Style Among Cultures?", she reported that children have their own learning styles that result "from innate tendencies and environmental experiences. Because cultural groups often share common values, the experiences of children growing up with those values are reflected in their classroom learning behaviors" (p. 1). Levinsohn (2007) conducted a comparative study regarding any significant differences in learning preferences and approaches between Chinese and European Trade students (p. 12). The research participants were Chinese and European students studying electrical and electronic trades in New Zealand. The results showed that Chinese students relied more on external regulation of their learning process than did students from European countries, who were more accustomed to student-centered teaching learning strategies.

The increasing amount of research focusing on the relationships between culture and learning styles will facilitate our understanding of the valuable contribution of cultural similarities and differences, in addition to bringing us a higher awareness of pedagogical methods and preferred learning styles throughout the world. It is our hope that culture-specific teaching learning philosophies, such as the Kindezi method of East Africa, which focuses on the nurturing of the whole person; research studies on the appropriate use and value of rote memorization; and the meaning and use of silence in teaching learning situations will be shared with teachers and learners worldwide.

Teaching methods used in one community or country may not work in other parts of the world. For example, in our teaching learning workshops in Ethiopia we soon learned not only that groups of participants or classes of students vary just like our participants and students in the United States, but also that there were some differences. The Ethiopian participants were more formal and respectful with each other and more reticent when responding to questions individually or volunteering to offer an opinion during the class than were American students. We soon learned that we needed to elicit their help in creating a teaching learning environment in which both teachers and participants could feel comfortable with longer moments of silence than we American teachers had been used to and in which a variety of personality types and learning styles could find their space.

EXHIBIT 3.2

A Reminder

Our first task in
     Approaching
          Another people
               Another culture
                    Another religion
Is to take off our shoes
     For the place we are
          Approaching is holy
     Else we may find ourselves
          Treading on another person's
               Dream.
                        —Anonymous

In the next section we further discuss the meaning and types of learning styles. The brief poem in Exhibit 3.2 reminds us to respect the differences, emphasize the similarities and honor the privileges we have to learn from people of many different cultures.

LEARNING STYLES

What Is a Learning Style?

Learning styles are important to understand. As a teacher, you create learning experiences and teaching materials for diverse students. Knowing how students learn, and knowing how you as a teacher learn, helps you to be responsive to students in a way that supports their learning.

A *learning style* has been defined as a particular set of behaviors and attitudes related to the teaching learning context. It is a student's consistent way of responding to and using stimuli in the context of learning. Romanelli et al. (2009) conducted a review of theory, application, and best practices with learning styles and offered their benchmark definition of *learning styles*: "characteristic cognitive [thinking], effective, and psychosocial behaviors that serve as relatively stable indicators of how learners perceive, interact with, and respond to the learning environment" (p. 1).

Teachers and students both bring their unique learning styles into the teaching learning environment. These learning styles may not match, leading to a clash. It is important for you as a teacher to understand learning styles so that you teach not only to your own learning style but also to the students' different learning styles, to increase their learning. The increase in cultural diversity throughout the world and the resultant mismatches in learning styles pose challenges for both students and teachers.

Brookfield (1990) stated that "On the face of it, if teachers wish to connect with as many students as possible, all they need to do is find out about the learning styles that students exhibit, and then adjust their teaching exercises and materials to the spread of styles that are revealed" (p. 67). He described several variables other than the student's preferred learning style that are important. The most important of these are the nature of the learning and the student's level of readiness, previous experiences and knowledge in the area, the student and the teacher's personalities, the personalities of other learners, the political ethos of the educational institutions, and the dominant values and traditions of the culture of which the student is a member.

Brookfield (1990) also claimed that teachers do not always need to adjust their practice to account for students' preferred learning styles; he also advocated doing the exact opposite. Understanding a student's learning style is helpful; however, instead of always affirming the preferred habitual, comfortable learning style, teachers might help their students by introducing them to new and alternative modes of learning (pp. 67–70).

The goal of this chapter is to help readers understand the reasons why they should be able to communicate the significance of the knowledge, skills, and attitudes required in the teaching learning process of health care worker students and to use information related to learning styles to support and increase students' learning.

There are several reasons to understand learning styles:

- It helps make teaching and learning more interactive.
- Teachers are better able to respond to students from diverse cultures.
- Teachers are better able to communicate significant information.
- It increases the students' retention of information.
- Students are diverse and learn differently.
- Without reflection on the practice of teaching, teachers are likely to teach as they learn.
- Teaching to different learning styles encourages innovation and creativity.
- Awareness of learning styles helps teachers enhance their methods of teaching and presentation.
- Understanding the benefit of using different learning styles encourages students to strengthen learning styles in which they are weak, leading to improved learning.

A learning style is a consistent way of responding to and using stimuli in the context of teaching and learning. Individuals develop a particular set of behaviors and attitudes toward learning. It is important that teachers understand that each learner approaches learning differently. The acts of seeing, hearing, feeling, and doing affect both student and teacher. Teaching and learning are interactive activities not only between teacher and student but also between student and student.

Learning Style Models

Today, there are several models of learning styles that use similar ideas to increase learning in many different settings, and with a groups of people with diverse learning preferences and styles. We present three models here: (a) the Myers–Briggs Type Indicator (MBTI) (Myers & McCaulley, 1986), (b) the Kolb Learning Cycle model (Kolb, 1984), and (c) the Felder–Silverman model (Felder & Silverman, 1988). Understanding learning styles and the importance of how students learn helps teachers develop instruction strategies that support students' multiple learning styles (Romanelli et al., 2009). As teachers reflect on their own preferred learning styles they become more attuned to the teaching learning strategies that will engage students with diverse learning preferences.

Myers–Briggs Type Indicator

The MBTI is often used in pedagogy and leadership training as well as many other fields where there is interest in learning to understand and appreciate ways of thinking and communicating with each other. The MBTI is based on Carl Jung's theory of personality types. The model consists of four pairs of indicators that can result in 16 different learning style types. Each pair indicates related though different attributes that have explanatory indicators along a continuum that ranges from more to less toward one of the attribute pairs. The four pairs include (a) Extraversion (E)–Introversion (I), (b) Sensing (S)–Intuition (N), (c) Thinking (T)–Feeling (F), and (d) Judging (J)–Perceptive (P).

Some persons may be much closer to the center of the Extraversion–Introversion continuum, whereas another person may be strongly extraverted or introverted. The MBTI contains a set of 126 questions, and the respondent's answers yield 1 of the 16 potential learning style types, such as ENTP (extravert, intuiting, thinking, perceiving) or IFSJ (introvert, feeling, sensing, judging). Myers and McCaulley (1986) provided a full description of the MBTI and how to use it.

EXTRAVERSION VERSUS INTROVERSION. Extraverts find energy in relating to people and in discussing and explaining ideas and concepts with others, whereas introverts find energy in their inner world of ideas, concepts, and abstractions. Extraverts prefer interaction with others and are action oriented. Introverts find energy in internal activities, such as formulating ideas and constructing frameworks. They can be sociable, but they need quiet time to recharge themselves. Extraverts, on the other hand, can do solitary work, but they recharge their batteries while relating to other people. Introverts want to understand the world; they are concentrators and reflective thinkers. They want to develop frameworks that integrate and/or connect the subject matter at hand. In contrast, extraverts learn by explaining to others, working in groups, engaging in projects, proposing change, and risking actions that have not been extensively investigated.

Teaching strategies for extraverts and introverts. Extraverts learn by explaining to others; this is how they know whether they understand the subject themselves. If they are unable to explain something to themselves or others, they realize they do not know the subject. Extraverts like working in groups on activities such as Think Aloud Paired Problem Solving (TAPPS) and the Nominal Group Method. Both of these active teaching learning strategies support learning through explaining and provide opportunities for introverted students to participate in small groups. The three roles of the teacher are to (a) pose a question and allow quiet time for students to think about the question, (b) divide the class into dyads or teams, and (c) critique responses and provide closure. Listeners can ask questions for clarification, disagree, or provide hints if the explainer becomes lost. The teacher critiques some of the answers and provides closure. This activity provides opportunities for asking questions, explaining, listening, sharing ideas, and critiquing responses.

Introverts approach learning in a different manner. They like to develop frameworks that integrate or connect the subject matter. To an introvert, disconnected pieces of information are not knowledge, but with a framework of facts the pieces become connected, and knowledge ensues. Teaching strategies for introverts include learning how to chunk and connect the knowledge. Three examples of how to do this would include (a) compare and contrast tables, (b) flow charts, and (c) concept mapping (see chap. 2, this volume, for a description of the use of content mapping).

SENSING VERSUS INTUITION. Some students choose to rely on their five senses—seeing, hearing, smelling, touching, and tasting—whereas others prefer to absorb information through the sixth sense: intuition. Sensing people are detailed oriented; they want facts and trust them. Where some people see patterns, others see randomness or chaos. Sensing students prefer organized and structured assignments and lectures (Brightman, 2010).

Teaching strategies for sensing and intuitive students. Three methods of organizing lectures for sensing students include (a) What Must Be Known (WMBK), (b) the application–theory–application method, and (c) the advanced organizer.

Teaching approaches such as WMBK, first present an application, problem, or mini-case. The student attempts to analyze and solve the problem by asking questions related to what must be known, without the benefit of the upcoming lecture during which theories and ideas will be discussed. The teacher then presents the lecture and applies it to the original case, involving students in the discussion.

What must be known includes the topics and the most essential general principles and questions related to the topic. First, what information or topics must be known so that students can achieve the outcomes/objectives that have been established? Second, students should continue to ask questions until all the information that is needed has been covered. The teacher can then present the interactive lecture by starting with the most basic questions and moving up to the most complex learning.

Another method that works for sensing students is the *application–theory–application* (A-T-A) method, or the *active teaching learning strategy*. Brightman

(2010) explained that with this method the teacher presents the application, such as a case, problem, or situation, before the lecture, and students attempt to analyze and solve an almost-solvable case/problem without the benefit of the theories or ideas. Sensing students are motivated to learn the material because this method answers the question of "why" the student needs to learn this material. The teacher encourages the students to continue to ask WMBK questions until the information is covered. After the class has struggled with the situation/problem, the theory and other relevant information are presented and discussed.

The third teaching strategy that is helpful to sensing students is the *advanced organizer*. An advanced organizer provides a mental scaffolding by starting with a familiar situation or setting on which the student can anchor the new knowledge. It is not an overview that would introduce students to new concepts. An advanced organizer taps into students' existing knowledge base and helps them connect the new information to existing information. The advanced organizer can be developed by asking oneself the following two questions:

1. At what educational level is the student, and what does the student know about the content to be taught?
2. What connections can be made between what is known and what is to be learned?

Brightman (2010) suggested that intuitive students, in contrast to sensing students, must have the "big picture" or an integrating framework to understand the subject. The big picture or a framework pulls the learning together and shows how it is related. Intuitive and sensing students respond to the *discovery method*, also known as the *"why" method*. Intuitive students can help sensing students to discover the theory, and sensing students can help intuitive students identify and manage the facts. Pairing sensing and intuitive students in a learning activity creates an opportunity for both to be exposed to different learning styles.

THINKING VERSUS FEELING. People who prefer to decide things impersonally, on the basis of analysis, logic, and cognitive principles, are considered to have learning preferences that lean toward the Thinking side of the Thinking–Feeling continuum, whereas people who tend to make decisions on the basis of human values and needs are considered to have learning preferences that fall closer to the Feeling end of the continuum. Thinking students value fairness and place great weight on objective criteria in making decisions. Students who use feelings to arrive at decisions value harmony and fairness and like working in groups. They are good at using persuasion and often are the facilitators in mediating differences in groups. They enjoy small group exercises such as TAPPS, and the Nominal Group Method.

Teaching strategies for thinking and feeling students. Teachers who want to appeal to thinking students' learning preferences should use clear and concise objectives and directions that are action oriented. They should also provide opportunities for students to solve problems using logic and analytical thinking. For feeling students, who tend to focus on human values and needs, teachers should use smaller group exercises, such as the Nominal Group Method and TAPPS. Both methods, as described by Brightman (2010), are active teaching learning strategies that have been used successfully in all 13 of the teaching learning workshops that were part of the Public Health Training Initiative in Ethiopia from 2001 to 2008. See Chapter 10 for description of the Public Health Training Initiative in Ethiopia. Brightman described the steps of these methods as follows:

1. **Nominal Group Method**
   - Teacher poses a question and provides quiet time for students.
   - The class is divided up into small groups called *teams*.
   - Each team member shares ideas with others in a round-robin fashion.
   - Teams discuss ideas and reach a group consensus.
   - Teacher critiques the teams' responses and provides closure.

2. **TAPPS**
   - Teacher poses a question and provides quiet time for students.
   - Teacher designates the explainer and listener within each student pair.
   - Explainers explain ideas to listeners.
   - Listeners can ask questions of clarification, disagree, or provide hints when explainers becomes lost.
   - Teacher critiques some explainers' answers and provides closure.

JUDGING VERSUS PERCEPTIVE. Judging people are planners; they are decisive and self-regulated (Brightman, 2010). They like to make quick decisions. They focus on completing the task, and they want to know only the essentials so they can take action quickly. They plan and then work their plan to meet the deadlines. In contrast, perceptive people tend to be curious and adaptable, and they enjoy the spontaneity of the moment. They tend to start many tasks, and want to know everything about each task, and thus they sometimes find it difficult to complete a task. They often postpone an assignment until the last minute. They see many options and thus seek more information until the last minute, completing the task or project in what they consider to be the nick of time.

Teaching strategies for judging and perceptive students. According to Brightman (2010), judging students tend to draw conclusions too quickly on a reading assignment, a project, or a case. Therefore, teachers need to use active teaching learning strategies that will help them take a second look. For example, when reviewing a case, a "second look" meeting may be set up. At this meeting one student takes on the role of adversary for the sake of pushing the understanding of the case further so that all aspects of the analysis are again reviewed. It is recommended that guidelines for a second-look meeting be included at the outset of the assignment. For perceptive students, who will often continue to seek information until the very last minute, Brightman suggested that a complex project or written assignment can be deconstructed into a series of smaller segments, each with its own deadline. This series of deadlines may help keep the perceptive students on target. This process can also provide the opportunity for continuous feedback, which in turn can have the added benefit of an opportunity for the students to improve their writing skills.

Understanding students' learning styles is important, because they may point to strategies that assist in helping students succeed. We have discussed the MBTI here as one example of an instrument that was designed to measure personality on the basis of prespecified personality types, and we have offered suggestions for active teaching learning strategies that may encourage different learning styles.

Kolb Learning Cycle Model

The Kolb learning cycle model is based on D. A. Kolb's (1984) experiential learning theory, which was discussed in chapter 2. Kolb theorized that people develop preferences for different learning styles much as they do for other styles, such as leadership or management. Kolb recommended that individuals need to understand the experiential learning model in order to understand and know what their own preferred learning style is. Kolb found that four combinations of perceiving and processing information determine four learning styles, based on four processes that must be present for learning to occur. The two types of learning preferences include (a) concrete experience or abstract conceptualization, in reference to how information is taken in, and (b) active experimentation or reflective observation, in reference to how information is internalized (Felder, 1996).

D. A. Kolb (2004) developed the Learning Styles Inventory (LSI), a set of questions, based on experiential learning theory, that help to identify the way people learn from experience (Kolb & Kolb, 2005). The LSI is similar to the MBTI in that the responses to the questions help determine the respondent's learning preferences according to four pairs of potential types. The classification scheme for four types of learners includes the following: (a) Accommodators (Concrete Experience–Active Experimentation), (b) Convergers (Abstract Conceptualization–Active Experimentation), (c) Assimilators (Abstract Conceptualization–Reflective Observation), and (d) Divergers (Concrete Experience–Reflective Observation). These learning styles represent the respondent's present preferences and should not be considered strengths and weaknesses. Some people may draw on more than one learning style, so it is important to avoid labeling and categorizing learners. However, "understanding one's own learning style can be helpful in improving learning speed, retention and enjoyment" (Kolb, 2004, p. 268).

TEACHING STRATEGIES FOR ACCOMMODATORS. Accommodators tend to be activists who learn best when they are completely involved. They are intuitive problem solvers and risk takers. Their preferred teaching learning activities are simulations and case studies.

TEACHING STRATEGIES FOR CONVERGERS. Convergers tend to be pragmatists who are interested in the practical application of ideas. They also enjoy problem solving and technical tasks, field work, and laboratory work.

TEACHING STRATEGIES FOR ASSIMILATORS. Assimilators are theorists who like to work with ideas and enjoy constructing models. They tend to be concise and logical, and they enjoy abstract concepts less than practical and human implications. Preferable teaching learning strategies for Assimilators are lecture and writing assignments.

TEACHING STRATEGIES FOR DIVERGERS. Divergers are reflective and tend to learn best by observation while making sense of experiences. They tend to be imaginative and interested in people and emotions. They, too, enjoy lectures and learn best by recording their thoughts and ideas in a learning log or journal.

D. A. Kolb's (2004) learning styles model has been used widely and compared and combined with other models, and continues to be one of the most useful because its emphasis is on learning from experience and it thus is applicable in many contexts, culturally and globally.

Felder–Silverman Learning Styles Model

This model, developed by Richard Felder and Linda Silverman (1988), incorporates five dimensions, two of which are similar to the MBTI and D. A. Kolb's (2004) Learning Styles Inventory. The perception or sensitive/intuitive dimension is very much like that of the MBTI and LSI. The processing (active/reflective) dimension is also in Kolb's model. The Felder–Silverman learning styles model incorporates five dimensions: (a) sensing/intuitive, (b) visual/verbal, (c) inductive/deductive, (d) active/reflective, and (e) sequential/global.

SENSING VERSUS INTUITIVE LEARNERS. Sensing learners tend to be practical and concrete, and they focus more on facts and tasks. Intuitive learners tend to be more conceptual and innovative, and they like to think about theories and their meanings.

VISUAL VERSUS VERBAL LEARNERS. Visual learners prefer visual representations, such as diagrams, charts, and pictures; verbal learners learn best with written and spoken explanations.

INDUCTIVE VERSUS DEDUCTIVE LEARNERS. Inductive learners enjoy presentations that move from specific to general, whereas deductive learners prefer presentations that proceed from general to specific. Deductive learners learn best when they can first see the "big picture."

ACTIVE VERSUS REFLECTIVE LEARNERS. Active learners need to try things in order to learn. They enjoy working with others. Reflective learners learn best by working alone with enough time to think things through by themselves.

SEQUENTIAL VERSUS GLOBAL LEARNERS. Sequential learners are linear, orderly thinkers who prefer to learn in small sequential steps. Global learners are holistic, systems-level thinkers who learn best in big leaps dealing with broad concepts.

These learning style models also present ways for teachers to understand learning. Being able to determine how students learn helps teachers select from a variety of teaching strategies that will match the students' learning styles, especially when students are having difficulties. Teachers realistically cannot match the learning styles of all students, but the use of a variety of different teaching learning strategies increases the opportunity for students to learn. At the end of this chapter, readers can complete Learning Activity 3.2 to determine the way they learn best. This information provides the opportunity for students to examine and discuss the ways they learn and to analyze the information and discuss their learning styles in a group setting. This information helps the teacher understand the students' learning styles and to use teaching strategies that promote student learning.

Implications for Teaching

Using a variety of active teaching strategies within the classroom increases the chance that students will have greater understanding and learning of the material at hand. Awareness of learning styles helps teachers enhance their methods of teaching and interacting with students to increase the students' learning. An understanding of different learning styles helps students recognize why they may be experiencing difficulty with the methods being used by a certain teacher. Understanding their own learning styles encourages students to develop and strengthen learning styles in which they are weak.

Teachers are not expected to develop different teaching methods for every student; however, striving to use a variety of teaching strategies has the potential to help students to broaden and/or change their learning styles. Using different styles makes teaching more rewarding, invigorates the teaching, and engages students. Exposing students to different learning styles encourages creativity and innovation. Students are not empty vessels that need to be filled but individuals who are to be engaged in the learning. Montgomery and Groat (1998) suggested that teaching and learning need to shift from the empty-vessel model to one of the dialogue–communal approaches, even in lecture classes. Classes need to include a variety of active teaching learning strategies that engage both students and teachers. Brookfield (1990) supported this idea of interspersing self-directed learning with collective cooperation in groups: "The principle of 'diversity in teaching' should be engraved on every teacher's heart" (p. 69).

As older individuals, immigrants, students with English as a second language, and cultural differences show up in classrooms in increasing numbers, there is a need to shift the emphasis on teaching and learning to active teaching strategies to engage students in dialogue that will lead to greater understanding of students and their learning-related interests, challenges, and desires. Life experiences from older students, culturally diverse students, and others enrich the classroom environment through sharing and dialogue. Teachers will need to build a "teaching toolkit" in which there are multiple active teaching learning strategies and approaches to address the different learning styles of students.

LEARNING ACTIVITY 3.1
CULTURE AND LEARNING

Question 1: How might knowledge about culture influence the selection and use of teaching and learning strategies?

Culture refers to the sum total of the lifeways of a group of people who share values, beliefs, and practices that are passed on from generation to generation and that change through time. For instance, in cultures such as most of those found in the United States, Canada, and Germany, where technology and efficiency are highly valued, cultural change is more rapid than in many African and Asian cultures, where human relationships and historical context have a higher value. In these cultures, change takes place more slowly.

Question 2: What are some examples in each level of culture that might relate to people learning about some public health or environmental health promotion concept that requires behavioral change?

Hidalgo (1993) suggested three levels of culture:

1. *Concrete:* The most visible and tangible artifacts, such as clothes, music, art, food, and games. Festivals and celebrations focus on these dimensions.
2. *Behavioral:* Practices that reflect values and define social and gender roles, languages spoken, and approaches to nonverbal communication. Behavioral aspects of culture include language, gender roles, family structure, political affiliation, and community organization.
3. *Symbolic:* Values and beliefs are often expressed in symbols and rituals.
4. Although symbolic meaning is often abstract, it is the key to how people define themselves in relation to each other, the world, and the universe. Symbolic expression includes value systems, religion, worldviews, customs, spirituality, morals, and ethics.

Question 3: What are the major cultural patterns in your own culture that might influence the way children learn? The way adults learn? What are the gender differences and expectations regarding learning?

There are many differences among families and individuals within a cultural group; these differences are referred to as *intracultural variation*. Nevertheless, there are recognizable patterns that give clues to the shared meanings and accepted actions within the group. These are known by the cultural group and are often misunderstood by persons outside the group. *Intercultural variation* refers to the differences between and among cultural groups.

Question 4: What methods of teaching and learning are used in your home? In your community?

Unless the teacher and the students are all from the same cultural group, there will be intercultural or transcultural differences. In most classrooms and learning situations there are multicultural challenges to consider. There may be perceived power differences among the cultures represented in the teaching learning context. There may be differences in how new health-related knowledge is incorporated into the community or family. There also may be differences in regard to who needs to sanction the knowledge that is imparted.

Question 5: How can you encourage your students to become more culturally open?

"A commitment to cultural openness is needed, as cultural boundaries are spanned during an interaction among persons, both clients and professional carers" (Wenger, 1999, p. 10). Cultural openness assumes promotion of cultural self-awareness and continuing development of transcultural teaching and learning skills.

In-Class Exercise 3.1: Looking at Your Cultural Interface

Pairs of students will discuss the following questions. Each pair of students will interview each other using the following questions. A large group discussion will follow.

1. **Identify the predominant cultural group to which you belong.**
2. **Describe two behaviors that generally characterize this group.**
3. **In what ways do you identify with these behaviors?**
4. **What characteristics of the group to which you belong do you most admire?**
5. **What characteristics of the group to which you belong do you not like?**
6. **Name a behavior from your culture that is health promoting.**
7. **Name a behavior from your culture that is a barrier to good health.**

From "Looking at Our Own Cultural Interface," by L. Chase and C. Dato, in L. S. Bermosk (Ed.), *An Adventure in Transcultural Communication and Health* (pp. 50–51), 1974, Honolulu: University of Hawaii Press.

In-Class Exercise 3.2: Cultural Learning and Critical Thinking

Divide the students or workshop participants into small groups for this assignment. If appropriate, form the groups according to health care discipline or parts of the city or country with which they are familiar, or some other viable grouping for this assignment.

Purpose: To use critical thinking principles in preparing students to enter a culture-specific village for community-based health care practice, such as health promotion activities.

Suggestions for the small groups: Choose a recorder and a reporter; read the scenario; answer all the items listed under "Setting the Stage for Cultural Learning"; choose only one of the critical thinking questions; discuss as a group; prepare a report to be given to the large group when everyone reconvenes.

Learning Activity 3.1   Culture and Learning (*Continued*)

Scenario:

Your university has instituted a policy for all departments to have students go to selected villages in suburban or rural areas during one semester of their program, where they will relate selected aspects of their discipline to the needs of the community.

For this exercise, imagine that you are preparing a group of students for field work in which they will be doing some aspect of health education within the village. How will you prepare them *culturally* for the fieldwork?

Guidelines:

Choose a discussion leader and a reporter. Use your previous experience and reflection on culture and learning to prepare a 5-minute presentation.

Setting the Stage for Cultural Learning

Answer Questions 1 through 4 and then choose one of the critical thinking questions.

1. Name the village and the culture or ethnic groups that live in the village.
2. Name the languages spoken in this village.
3. Name a culture marker for each of the three levels of culture listed in Learning Activity 3.1 that are relevant to health promotion or disease prevention.
4. Describe the chosen culture marker in terms of its relevance for that village.

Using Critical Thinking and Cultural Openness Concepts

1. *Examining our beliefs in light of facts and lived experiences guides us in becoming aware of underlying assumptions.* What are some of the underlying assumptions about this cultural group? How will you help students become aware of their cultural assumptions about this cultural group?
2. *An attitude of openness sets the tone for inquiry.* How will you prepare students to understand themselves culturally? How will you help them discover their own inquiry methods that honor and respect a culture different from their own?
3. *Recognizing patterns opens the way for analysis of differences and understanding of a situation.* What are some patterns that may indicate the specific health education that could be useful in this village?
4. *Critical thinking involves the pursuit of meaning and communication of meanings that are understood by the cultural group and the health professionals.* What does health or healing mean to people of this culture? How will your students learn the cultural meanings of health and healing from the villagers?
5. *Metaphors and symbols used by cultures to explain life and other phenomena from their perspective are valuable sources of information needed for cultural understanding.* How will you guide your students in learning about metaphors and symbols related to health and illness so that they can use this knowledge in

the health education they will do in the village? What are the proverbs or traditional stories related to health or illness in this culture?

6. *Critical thinking and clinical decision making are similar in that both are searching for creative solutions in difficult situations.* How will you guide your students in deciding the what, where, when, and how they will do health education in this village? How will they incorporate the cultural meanings of health and healing related to this village in their teaching learning plan?

LEARNING ACTIVITY 3.2

LEARNING STYLES

HOW DO PEOPLE LEARN?

Overview

Learning styles are important to understand. As a teacher, one creates learning experiences and teaching materials for students. Knowing how students learn, and how you as a teacher learn, influences your teaching and the success of students. This learning activity provides information on learning styles, an approach to determining learning styles, and an opportunity to think about your own learning style preferences and how they impact you as student and/or teacher.

Directions

Read the following references.

1. *Georgia State University Master Teacher Program* (Brightman, 2010): http://www2 .gsu.edu/~dschjb/wwwmbti.html
2. *Disabilities, Opportunities, Internetworking and Technology*: http://www.washington .edu/doit/TeamN/learn.html

As you read the articles, write down questions that come to mind. Complete the Learning Styles Questionnaire (presented next) and turn it in to the teacher. Discussion will focus on the information of the learning styles of the class and their implications for teaching and learning.

LEARNING STYLES QUESTIONNAIRE

Directions

Respond to the following questions. Read the information on learning styles as listed in the references. Compare your answers with the information on learning styles to see if you can identify your learning styles. Break into pairs and discuss your answers. Do you know what learning style you use most often?

1. The way I learn best is: _____
2. Do you consider yourself an outgoing person or a shy person?
3. Do you prefer doing something or thinking about something?
4. Which is easier for you to learn: concrete information, such as facts, or abstract information, such as ideas, concepts, and relationships?
5. Do you prefer to make decisions on the basis of your thinking or on the basis of your feelings?
6. Do you prefer to focus on completing the task, wanting only the essentials, or are you curious, adaptable, and spontaneous?
7. Do you rely on your senses (seeing, hearing, feeling, smelling, taste),or do you trust your feelings and intuition?

REFERENCES

Brightman, H. J. (2010). *Georgia State University Master Teacher Program*. Retrieved from http://www2.gsu.edu/~dschjb/wwwmbti.html

Brookfield, S. D. (1990). *The skillful teacher*. San Francisco, CA: Jossey-Bass.

De Vita, G. D. (2001). Learning styles, culture and inclusive instruction in the multicultural classroom: A business and management perspective. *Innovations in Education & Teaching International, 38,* 165–174.

Felder, R. M. (1996). Matters of style. *ASEE Prism, 6*(4), 18–23. Retrieved from http://www4.ncsu.edu/unity/lockers/users/f/felder/public/Papers/LS-Prism.htm

Felder, R. M., & Silverman, L. K. (1988). Learning and teaching styles in engineering education. *Engineering Education, 78,* 674–681. Retrieved from http://www4.ncsu.edu/unity/lockers/users/f/felder/public/Papers/LS-1988.pdf

Fierro, D. (1997). *Is there a difference in learning style among cultures?* Retrieved from ERIC database. (ED415974)

Grasha, A. F. (1990). Using traditional versus naturalistic approaches to assessing learning styles in college teaching. *Journal of Excellence in College Teaching, 1,* 23–38.

Gunderson, G. R. (2004). *Boundary leaders: Leadership skills for people of faith*. Minneapolis, MN: Fortress Press.

Hall, E. T. (1976). *Beyond culture*. Garden City, NY: Anchor Press/Doubleday.

Hildago, N. (1993). Multicultural teacher introspection. In T. Perry & J. Fraser (Eds.), *Freedom's plow: Teaching in a multicultural classroom* (pp. 99–105). New York, NY: Routledge.

Kolb, A. Y., & Kolb, D. A. (2005). *The Kolb Learning Styles Inventory—Version 3.1: 2005 technical specifications*. Retrieved from http://www.learningfromexperience.com/images/uploads/Tech_spec_LSI.pdf

Kolb, D. A. (1984). *Experiential learning: Experience as a source of learning and development*. Englewood Cliffs, NJ: Prentice Hall.

Kolb, D. A. (2004). Learning Style Inventory. In A. Lowry & P. Hood (Eds.), *The power of the 2 × 2 matrix* (pp. 267–268). San Francisco, CA: Jossey-Bass.

Leininger, M. M. (1991). *Culture care diversity and universality: Theory of nursing*. New York, NY: National League for Nursing.

Levinsohn, K. R. (2007). Cultural differences and learning styles of Chinese and European Trades students. *Institute for Learning Styles Journal, 1,* 12–22.

Montgomery, S. M., & Groat, L. N. (1998). *Student learning styles and their implications for teaching*. Occasional Paper No. 10, Center for Research on Learning and Teaching, University of Michigan. Retrieved from http://www.crlt.umich.edu/publinks/CRLT_no10.pdf

Myers, I. B., & McCaulley, M. H. (1986). *Manual: A guide to the development and use of the Myers–Briggs Type Indicator* (2nd ed.). Palo Alto, CA: Consulting Psychologists Press.

Palmer, P. J. (1998). *The courage to teach: Exploring the inner landscape of a teacher's life*. San Francisco, CA: Jossey-Bass.

Reagan, T. (2005). *Non-Western educational traditions: Indigenous approaches to educational thought and practice* (3rd ed.). Mahwah, NJ: Erlbaum.

Romanelli, F., Bird, E., & Ryan, M. (2009). Learning styles: A review of theory, application, and best practices. *American Journal of Pharmaceutical Education, 73,* 1–5.

Wenger, A. F. Z. (1991). The role of context in culture-specific care. In P. L. Chinn (Ed.), *Anthology on caring* (pp. 95–110). New York, NY: National League for Nursing.

Wenger, A. F. Z. (1993). Cultural meaning of symptoms. *Holistic Nursing Practice, 7,* 22–35.

Wenger, A. F. Z. (1998). Cultural openness, social justice, global awareness: Promoting transcultural nursing with unity in a diverse world. In P. Merilainen & K. Vehvilainen-Julkunen (Eds.), *Transcultural nursing—Global unifier of care, facing diversity with unity* (pp. 162–168). Kuopio, Finland: Kuopio University Publications.

Wenger, A. F. Z. (1999). Cultural openness: Intrinsic to human care. *Journal of Transcultural Nursing, 10,* 10.

4

Teaching in Classroom Settings

Teaching in a classroom setting is the most traditional sort of education one may consider. In a low-resource environment, the classroom setting may be everything from a modern university to a semicircle of students under a nearby shade tree. A classroom may also be defined as any setting where patients are not present. However, although classroom settings may vary wildly across domains, resources, and cultures, established techniques used within a classroom contain many similarities.

In this chapter we cover four main active teaching learning strategies that are effective in a classroom setting: (a) storytelling, (b) reflection, (c) lecture, and (d) critical thinking. These methods of teaching and learning are both traditional and adaptable to any setting.

STORYTELLING AND REFLECTION

Storytelling to Impart Knowledge

Often, a *story* is defined as anything that can be told or recounted—a tale of a happening that comprises a connected series of occurrences that may be true or false. Storytelling is an ancient teaching strategy and a method of organizing and communicating knowledge in a way that, if performed effectually, is entertaining to the listener. Telling a story is a valuable way to communicate integrity of knowledge, or to connect information to develop meaning and understanding. Understanding what gives meanings to stories, and how you as a teacher can enhance the connectivity among stories related to teaching, health promotion, and disease prevention, is an important role in the classroom.

Parents tell children stories that illustrate lessons to be learned, hold meanings, and pass on history; teachers tell stories to students that also illustrate lessons to be learned, hold meanings, and pass on knowledge. Storytelling is a teaching learning strategy that helps one describe and clarify experiences and reflect and gain different perspectives; it is purposeful and goal directed, and it requires few resources and little or no expense. Stories help to describe and clarify situations and experiences by examining different perspectives, information, values, and beliefs. Stories often trigger memories of one's own experiences and provide opportunities to reflect on situations for better understanding. In short, storytelling is an art, and it has power as a vital teaching tool that leads to understanding because it

- helps to describe and clarify our experiences,
- requires one to reflect and gain different perspectives,
- is purposeful and goal directed, and
- provides clues to our values and beliefs based on our experiences.

Stories have been used as a teaching tool with children so that wisdom and lessons of survival can be passed on to the next generation. Stories also can be effectively used in education and public health. The meanings of various stories used in the education of health professionals are derived from the culture of a storyteller and his or her audience. Stories can be true, fictional, or a mixture of both, but the purpose of storytelling is the same: to impart a lesson or knowledge in a way that is engaging and meaningful to the listener.

Because culture is the glue that maintains the connections between families, groups, and societies, and because cultural knowledge and the competency of health professionals often impact the quality and safety of health care, it is important to take culture into account while storytelling. Teachers have opportunities to promote cultural knowledge and competencies while educating nurses and other health professionals, and they should consider culture prominently when developing stories for use in the classroom. It is essential for instructors to develop cross-cultural communication skills when working with or telling stories to multicultural students, mostly to avoid pitfalls such as stereotyping, misuse of language registers, misunderstanding taboos, inconsiderate gestures, inappropriate body language, or behavior stereotyping (see chap. 3, this volume, for more information on culture).

Reflection for Learning

Reflection is a mental process that people use every day, and one's ability to reflect is developed out of personal and professional experiences. Reflection allows one to critique, test, and make meaning out of experiences. It is an active, persistent, and careful consideration of any belief or supposed form of knowledge in the light of evidence that supports it. Like storytelling, reflection can be used in any setting and, used effectively, is an inexpensive teaching learning strategy.

Reflection is sometimes referred to as a process that occurs internally and in isolation. Boud, Keogh, and Walker (1985) stated that "reflection in the context of learning" is a generic phrase for those intellectual and affective activities in which individuals engage to explore their experiences, leading to new understandings and appreciations (p. 19). This understanding will in turn link reflection to experience. Like Boud et al., Boyd and Fales (1983) also linked reflection to experience and offered a useful definition of reflection as a process of internally examining an issue of concern, triggered by an experience, that creates and clarifies meaning in terms of the self and that results in a changed conceptual perspective or a different way of knowing and understanding the world.

Boud et al.'s (1985) model of reflection in learning consists of two components: (a) the experience and (b) the reflective activity. They defined *experience* as the total response of a person to a situation or event: what he or she thinks, feels, does, and concludes at the time and immediately thereafter. They contended that the experience is followed by a processing phase of reflection. Reflection is an important human activity in which people recapture their experience, think about it, mull it over, and evaluate it. In Boud et al.'s view, one of the most important ways to enhance learning is to strengthen the link between experience and the reflective activity that follows it. When using reflection in educational settings, teachers should plan consciously for the reflective phase, because it is often overlooked and undervalued.

Boud et al. (1985) went on to state that reflection consists of an active, persistent, and careful consideration of a belief, action, or situation so that one can understand and determine meaning. The act of reflection allows students to make connections between classroom discussion and practical experience in the real world without the demands and responsibilities of practice. Encouraging students to share their experiences through storytelling is a positive way to increase reflection and learning. As an active teaching learning strategy, reflection helps students to be engaged and to organize information; facilitates knowledge recollection; and enhances discussion, problem posing, and problem solving. Reflection has distinct benefits for the teacher, too. According to Boud et al., reflection can lead to the following accomplishments:

- Acquiring technical competence as a teacher and practitioner
- Being able to analyze one's own teaching and clinical practice and the practice of others
- Increasing one's awareness of ethical and moral choices inherent to teaching and learning
- Being sensitive to the diversity of students' backgrounds, characteristics, and abilities
- Teaching students to use reflection as a learning tool

Boud et al. (1985) also detailed three key assumptions regarding reflection in learning:

1. Only learners themselves can learn, and only they can reflect on their own experiences.
2. Although facilitators can access learners' thoughts by a variety of methods at a very basic level, learners have complete control in a teaching learning situation by choosing what they are willing to share.

3. Reflection is pursued with intent; it is a purposive activity directed toward a goal. The reflective process is a complex one in which both feeling and thinking are closely interrelated and interactive.

Boud et al. (1985) also suggested that, in any learning experience, three stages are present and require different types of reflection: (a) preparation, (b) engagement, and (c) processing. In the *preparation* phase, learners deal with the anticipation of the experience, reflecting perhaps on what might be expected of them and what contribution they might make. In the *engagement* phase, the actual experience, learners' reflections usually include recognition of the disparity between what they have learned in the classroom and what they experience in the field. The final phase, *processing*, occurs after the field experience and involves reflecting on the experience to make sense of and get meaning from it.

Boud et al. (1985) identified three elements as being central to this reflective process:

1. **Returning to the experience.** This element involves recalling the important aspects of the experience. It is descriptive in nature and requires that the learner recall what actually occurred as accurately as possible. The simple recollection of an event can develop insight. As we witness the events again, they become available to us to reconsider and examine afresh; we realize what we were feeling and what responses prompted us to act as we did (Boud et al., 1985, p. 27). The description itself should be as free from judgment and interpretations as possible.
2. **Attending to feelings.** This element involves the learner consciously recalling positive and negative feelings that he or she may have encountered during the experience. Boud et al. recommended that positive feelings be used to assist in pursuing what otherwise might be a very challenging situation.
3. **Reevaluating the experience.** During this element of the reflection process the experience is reexamined in light of the learner's intent, while associating new knowledge with what was already known and integrating this new knowledge into the learner's conceptual framework. Boud et al. described four subelements within the process of reevaluation:
   a. **Association.** *Association* is the connecting of the ideas and feelings that were a part of the original experience with those that have occurred during reflection. Through this process we may come to realize that our previous attitudes are no longer consistent with our new understanding.
   b. **Integration.** During this aspect of reevaluating the experience, the process of discrimination helps us determine what is meaningful to us. Two processes are involved in this aspect: (a) searching for the nature of drawing conclusions and (b) arriving at insights. During reevaluation the individual experiences a merging, or creative synthesis, of the information previously taken in with the formation of a new solution or change in the self.

c. **Validation.** In this aspect, learners begin to test their new understandings for consistency with their existing knowledge and beliefs. If discrepancies appear, the situation needs to be reassessed so the learner can decide on what basis to proceed. Rehearsal is a useful strategy to use in the validation aspect.

d. **Appropriation.** *Appropriation* involves the learner owning the new information in a personal way. Strong emotions are involved in this process, and the individual is affected deeply by the learning. This aspect does not occur in all instances of reevaluating an experience.

Storytelling and Reflection Used Together

Stories can arise from the practical experiences of both the teacher and student, bringing into the classroom real world experience as lived by the storyteller, which in turn can provide information and learning about a particular scenario. Storytelling and reflection as teaching strategies bring the real world into the classroom, where students and teacher reflect with an active, purpose-oriented process to examine the story for learning and meaning. This creates a link between the classroom and clinical learning for health profession students.

Reflection and learning do not happen *to* you or *for* you. For true reflection to occur within a student, he or she must participate in the classroom activities. Reflections may be shared, or they may be private. Reflection may be described as talking to yourself "in your head." The processes involved in reflecting on a story or an experience can be very personal and indicative of what you think you have learned and what it means to you. Reflection allows you time to comprehend the meanings of a lesson or situation and to clarify misconceptions.

Storytelling as a classroom activity encourages reflection, as long as the story emphasizes accuracy, description, and a multifaceted examination of information. For effective reflection, a story must also describe the environment in which the incident/event occurred, who was involved, and the outcomes or changes that happened as a result of any interventions.

LECTURE

Lecture has been a part of educational experiences for decades and is therefore very familiar to teachers and students. Teachers and students often have a picture or image of how a class works: The professor talks, and the students listen. Although in the past lecture has been the teaching method used most frequently, it is not necessarily the most effective for learning. Lecture is inexpensive and flexible, and it offers a way of teaching content when other resources are not available.

TABLE 4.1		
TYPES OF LECTURES		
Expository	**Lecture–Recitation**	**Interactive**
What students think of most often as a lecture: The teacher talks, and the students listen. The teacher talks most of the time, and students ask few questions.	Encourages greater student participation. The teacher does most of the talking but stops, asks questions, or requests that students read material. Interactions are in the form of teacher to class, teacher to individual student, or individual student to teacher.	Encourages student-to-student interactions. Teacher gives mini-lectures, and students break into small groups for discussion. The teacher may then deliver another mini-lecture.

Source: Brightman (2010).

Being an effective lecturer requires good communication skills and knowing how to include students in discussion for an active teaching learning session (Table 4.1). Keeping students' attention is always a challenge during a lecture, but it is rewarding when it happens. The following sections focus on how to plan and present an effective lecture.

How to Plan a Lecture

Every lecture has three components: (a) an introduction, (b) a body, and (c) a conclusion. There is an old American adage that perfectly states how a lecture should be structured: "Tell them what you are going to tell them, tell them, and then tell them what you told them."

Lecture Introduction

A lecture's introduction provides information on what is to be covered in the lecture and how the lecture is structured. The introduction serves as an "advance organizer" and prepares the students for the lecture. Often, an outline of the lecture content is helpful to give students so they can follow along with the teacher. The introduction gives the instructor the opportunity to gain the students' attention by sharing the topic of the lecture, explaining why it is important, and describing the anticipated outcomes. Within the introduction, techniques such as providing statistics and storytelling stimulate the students' interest in hearing more on the topic. It's a good idea to use stories and scenarios in the introduction, such as providing evidence why the topic is important and linking the material to other lectures on the topic, to arouse the students' attention. Sharing the topic and the outcomes/objectives of the lecture in the beginning prepares the students for identifying the major learning that is to occur. A discussion outline, overview, and/or desired outcomes within a lecture introduction are helpful to students so they can follow the discussion and organize their notes.

Lecture Body

The body of a lecture covers the major points to be learned. Teaching strategies that require student participation in the lecture or activity are helpful because the listeners are then able to follow along and to organize their learning. The lecture body is the longest part, and it contains the majority of the information that is to be imparted to the students. It is in the body that statistics, diagrams, major points of knowledge, and lessons learned are presented. During a lecture, it is often permissible to allow the students to ask clarifying questions, which encourages participation and engagement and allows the instructor to know whether the students are following along with the direction of the discussion.

Lecture Conclusion

In the lecture conclusion, the instructor summarizes the body of the lecture and succinctly reviews the major points of information. The instructor should link the conclusion back to the introduction by reviewing the outline of what was discussed and explaining how the information was useful or important for the students to know and understand. Often a lecture conclusion is short, but it can be as long as necessary to review all the major points of learning that the students are expected to take away from the teaching learning session. Clarification questions can also be asked during the conclusion. After the conclusion, the instructor should continue the learning process by asking direct questions related to the body of the lecture so that students can solidify the knowledge they have gained.

Lecture as an Active Teaching Learning Strategy

Lecture has been the major tool in educational settings for many years, and some teachers avoid active teaching learning strategies because they believe they reduce the time that is available for lecture. McKeachie, Pintrich, Lin, Smith, and Sharma (1990) demonstrated that much is known about how learning happens and that not much learning occurs in the classroom unless students are actively involved. Silberman (1996) stated that content coverage can occur in small groups without sacrificing quality or quantity of knowledge.

Students who are familiar with lecture from earlier educational experiences can feel frustrated when faced with other teaching learning strategies in the classroom. Because of the familiarity and traditional use of lecture in a classroom setting, students might complain if teachers do not lecture, because the students may feel their expectations are not being met; they might want the teacher to "Tell me what I need to know, and don't make me search for it." Because of students' preference for lecture in some classrooms and environments, the low cost of lecture when there are limited resources for education in the classroom setting, and the ability to make a lecture engaging, it is possible to use a lecture as an active teaching learning strategy.

The following list describes six commonly used active teaching learning strategies that teachers can incorporate into a lecture discussion. These strategies can also serve as classroom assessment techniques, because they allow the teacher to assess students' understanding. These strategies shift responsibility for engagement to students and allow them to do most of the work by using their brains, studying ideas, and problem solving.

1. **Think–Pair–Share.** Introduced by Lyman (1981), this method is often recommended for teachers who are beginning to explore interactive collaborative learning situations. A question, dilemma, or problem is posed by the instructor, and students think about assumptions made, errors, ethical issues, or other topics. Students then pair with a partner to compare answers and prepare a joint response.
2. **Short writes.** This is a strategy that can be used at the end of a lecture to stimulate discussion. Each student is given a 4 × 6-inch card, or piece of paper, and is asked to write a summary of the main points covered during the lecture. Students may also relate the lecture to the overall goals of the course. After writing their observations, students should be paired to discuss what they learned from the lecture. After their small group discussion, students then rewrite their overall observations on the lecture on the other side of the card or piece of paper, for approximately 2 minutes, and submit the card to the instructor as they leave the class session. Information from students' observations can aid the instructor in preparing their next lecture or class discussion on the topic.
3. **Application cards.** DeYoung (2003) described this technique as an opportunity for students to apply theoretical knowledge and provide the teacher with timely feedback. After the teacher describes a theory or body of knowledge, students write down a possible application of that knowledge. The teacher can then read the best examples and clarify issues related to the worst.
4. **Paraphrasing.** This strategy can be particularly helpful to health care workers because they often have to paraphrase or "translate" often-complex medical terms into more commonly understood language. The student simply paraphrases something he or she has just learned. This can be done by calling on the student to speak openly to the class, or it can be done in pairs, with a student pair volunteering their own "translation."
5. **Think Aloud Paired Problem Solving.** This collaborative problem-solving technique has been called the most powerful classroom instructional strategy to promote understanding of a lecture (Felder & Brent, 2003). Students work in pairs to solve problems. One student is the "Listener," and the other is the "Problem Solver." The Problem Solver analyzes the problem, finds the assumptions being made, explains an observation, and finds errors or answers to other questions. In the next activity, the Problem Solver and Listener switch

roles. The new Problem Solver then reads the problem out loud and goes through the solution or answer, while the new Listener listens to each step.

6. **Strategies to facilitate small group work.** Small group (4–6 members) work is increasingly being used with case methods, discussion, course content, and other active teaching learning strategies, particularly after students attend a lecture. Providing students with structure and tips for being successful in small group work leads to more success in their learning. Including tips on effective communication styles to students sets up opportunities in which all group members have a chance to learn how to be a contributing member in small groups and to voice their opinions. The instructor should encourage group members to be culturally sensitive to one another, and to not stereotype each other, because this may hamper discussion. The instructor should develop a structure or process to guide communication, such as selecting topics for discussion that provide opportunities for each group member to participate or speak. The instructor also should provide information on effective communication and listening skills. Negative behaviors that affect group work include students not listening to each other, labeling one another, and not allowing multiple perspectives to be heard. Encouragement by the instructor of clear, appropriate communication is essential to successful group work that can inform and complement a classroom lecture.

CRITICAL THINKING

Health professionals work in situations in which they must think critically in order to provide safe and competent care. Educating health workers to be critical thinkers is a challenge for teachers and instructors. Other terms have been used to describe the process of critical thinking. Dewey (1933) used the term *reflective thinking* and identified three elements in the process: (a) a desire to address the problem; (b) acceptance that the problem needs to be solved, and (c) solving the problem. Bandman and Bandman (1995) focused on the role of reasoning in critical thinking. Facione (2010) describes critical thinking, based upon the consensus of a national panel of experts, as being able to interpret, analyze, evaluate, and make inferences. A critical thinker can also explain why and how they arrive at a judgment. In addition, they apply critical thinking to themselves for self improvement.

In the field of health care, the scientific method is one well-known process that leads to making appropriate decisions through critical thinking. Bradshaw and Lowenstein (2011) stated that critical thinking is needed today in all health care settings, which are usually busy and situated in complex, high-tech environments. In low-resource environments with limited resources and few emergency support facilities, critical thinking is definitely a needed skill. Siegel (1980) stated that critical thinking serves the following three functions: (a) It facilitates students' self-sufficiency and autonomy, (b) it helps students reason and make judgments, and (c) it allows students to take action on the basis of a reasonable assessment.

Benner, Sutphen, Leonard, and Day (2010), in their book *Educating Nurses: A Call for Radical Transformation*, returned to Dewey's (1933) mandate to reflect on experience, which leads to the formation of pre- and postclinical deliberations on critical thinking found in nursing education today. Active teaching learning strategies used in the education of health professionals emphasize the importance of critical thinking. Teaching students in the health care profession to become critical thinkers is thus an essential part of their preparation.

Definitions of *Critical Thinking*

Frank Smith (1990), in his book *To Think*, provided a list of verbs that are important to use when talking about thinking. Smith (1990, p. 1) provides a list of 77 words that refer to thinking. He believes that words are clues to the things that people believe to be important. His list of words related to thinking include analyze, assert, conceptualize, hypothesize, postulate, conceptualize, along with many others related to thinking. These action verbs are similar to the verbs that teachers use to write behavioral objectives. In essence, these verbs focus not on the brain but on what people are doing. For many years, teachers focused on behavioral objectives and not so much on the quality of thinking. Instructors talked about critical thinking; however, the focus was not on the student's brain but on what the student is able to do. Instructors could determine the student's ability to perform a skill at a certain level, but not know that student's level of knowledge. All humans think; it is part of human nature. The problem is that much of our thinking, left to itself, becomes biased, distorted, partially informed, and prejudiced. The quality of our lives, what we produce, learn, and accomplish, depends on our thinking. Thinking can be cultivated, educated, and improved. Benner et al. (2010) highlighted the need for teachers in the health care field to shift to an emphasis on clinical reasoning and multiple ways of thinking, including critical thinking, in the training of health care professionals.

Bandman and Bandman (1995) presented three models of teaching and learning about critical thinking in nursing: (a) feelings, (b) vision, and (c) examination. These are essential to health workers so that they might gather data and information on patients. Feelings might derive from instinctual reactions or impressions or from evidence-based data. Understanding these feelings and their source can help a health professional better understand the patient and situation. However, along with feelings comes the need for vision and examination so that one understands what to do with the information. The desired outcome for both the health care professional and the patient is to arrive at a hypothesis about the situation that they can explore or test to assist in critical decision making.

Bradshaw and Lowenstein (2011) traced the history of critical thinking from Dewey (1933) to Watson and Glaser (1980), Ennis (1985) and Paul (1993) to the most recent definition of critical thinking developed by the American Philosophical Association (Facione, 1990).

> The American Philosophical Association described a critical thinker as habitually inquisitive, well-informed, trustful of reason, open-minded, flexible, fair-minded in evaluation, honest in facing personal biases, prudent in making judgments, willing to reconsider, clear about issues, orderly in complex matters, diligent in seeking relevant information, reasonable in the selection of criteria, focused in inquiry, and persistent in seeking results which are as precise as the subject and circumstance of inquiry permit. (p. 3)

Selected Elements of Critical Thinking

There are several elements of critical thinking development of which an instructor must be aware that will help them guide their students to understand.

Awareness of Underlying Assumptions

An *assumption* is a belief that is held as truth without supportive information on data. Education and critical thinking force one to examine beliefs in light of facts and lived experiences and to be clear and unambiguous. Critical thinking helps us simplify our beliefs and recognize the need for flexibility in light of new thoughts, evidence, information, and reflection (Dewey, 1933). People make assumptions, and action often precedes analytic thought rather than resulting from it. Identifying and challenging assumptions are central to critical thinking and clinical judgment in practice. The ability to recognize assumptions being made in one's work as a health professional is essential to developing expertise in practice.

Inquiry Methods

An attitude of openness by a health care professional sets the tone for inquiry. Openness is a quality in a person that allows recognition of differences and seeks an understanding of problems, situations, beliefs, and possible solutions. The way a health care professional views a situation sets the stage for action. The following are some examples of questions that instructors can ask themselves to determine the openness of a situation:

- What is the mindset that I, as the instructor, as well as the students, bring to a situation?
- To what degree do teachers and students distort or misinterpret situations in order to fit a predetermined mindset?
- How open are teachers to seeing what really exists or works?
- How willing are students, instructors, and practitioners willing to listen to and hear each other's views, thoughts, and ideas that may be different from our own?

Inquiring minds seek answers, information, and solutions. Inquiry methods such as the ones just listed are essential to all types of education and to successful functioning in a rapidly changing world and health care system. Inquiry will be a constant process for health professionals. Recognizing that what you learn today will be obsolete in 1 to 2 years, or less, emphasizes the importance of developing your personal inquiry methods and/or knowing how you learn best.

Questioning

Have you heard the slogan "Question authority"? Closely related to inquiry methods is the technique of raising questions. A young child learns about his or her world through questioning. A toddler's "Why . . .?" questions elicit information and understanding. Questioning is crucial to eliciting information about and understanding different perspectives, to distinguishing facts from assumptions, to making decisions about what to believe and what not to believe, to gathering data that are needed to understand situations and their contexts, to understanding existing relationships and power issues, to critiquing readings and other media, and to questioning what one learns about a given subject. Skepticism is healthy and leads one to ask appropriate questions. Raising questions requires one to think about a given topic or the situation. If one is not raising questions, then one must ask "Are you thinking"?

Many challenges and scenarios will require health care professionals to engage in questioning, and teaching health care students to explore their environments through questioning will serve them well as practitioners, especially in low-resource countries. Health care workers will play key roles in the changing future of health delivery. As an instructor, encourage your students to begin asking questions about where changes will take place, how one might improve the quality of health care, how one serves a culturally diverse population, and what an individual health care professional's role will be within a delivery system.

Recognizing Patterns

Have you ever suddenly become aware that something seems to be repeating itself over and over? You are not sure what it is, but you recognize that something is happening repeatedly. *Pattern recognition* is the perceptual ability that enables humans to recognize configurations and relationships without analytically specifying the components of the patterns. What is it that seems to occur frequently? What are you aware of about a situation you have encountered that seems repetitive? Once patterns are recognized, they can then be analyzed and studied so that we can understand and clarify what is happening. Recognizing patterns brings order to what may have seemed like chaos. It provides a way of tying together, in meaningful ways, events that occur over time.

Assigning Meaning

What is *meaning*? The word itself has several definitions. Bandman and Bandman (1995) offered four definitions or descriptions of *meaning*. First, it is an indication or an implication of a state of affairs. An example of this is that rain may lead to an excellent crop for farmers, or it may ruin a celebratory event, or cause a flood. Cues or clues offer possibility of meanings in a given context. A second definition of *meaning* is in asking for cause and effect, as in "What do those raised spots on the child's body mean?" A third definition refers to intent or purpose. An example of this may be when one nurse asks another what she meant when she told the patient to ignore the physician's orders. A fourth definition refers to the significance of implications, such as with the question "What does it mean to be involved with a dying patient?" Each of us search for meaning in our lives. Critical thinking provides the tools to help us understand the meanings of scenarios. To engage in critical thinking is to pursue meaning and to communicate meanings in ways that are clear, concise, and understandable. In the process of assigning meaning one will use knowledge gained, attitudes, values, morality, and one's own experiences.

Recognizing Symbols

Symbols, and their respective cultural meanings, provide ways to define, describe, and relate to the world around us. Connections to symbols are used to think about and anchor us to life experiences. Metaphorical thinking is based on symbols. An example of a metaphor is "A rolling stone gathers no moss." This metaphor means that keeping active keeps the brain sharp. Metaphor and symbols used by various cultures to explain life and phenomena from their perspectives are valuable sources of information to health care workers, and an instructor should emphasize that health care professionals need to recognize symbols when interviewing or examining their patients.

Making Judgments and Decisions

Judgments and decisions are the ultimate outcomes of critical thinking. A desire to be a good practitioner leads one to search for concrete answers to many difficult situations in which creative solutions are needed. Critical thinking approaches to practice are based on hypotheses that may or may not prove to be useful after being tested. There are similarities between the critical thinking process and clinical decision making, based on how one determines their judgments. Discussion of this process and how it can best serve a health care professional is an important topic for an instructor to cover in a classroom setting.

LEARNING ACTIVITY 4.1

USING STORYTELLING AND REFLECTION IN PLANNING A LECTURE

OVERVIEW

Storytelling is a method of organizing and communicating knowledge. It is a valuable way to communicate the integrity of knowledge or to connect information to develop meaning. Storytelling is an art, and it has power as a vital teaching tool because it describes and clarifies experiences, requires reflection to gain different perspectives, is purposeful and goal directed, and provides clues to our values and beliefs. In this learning activity we discuss what gives meanings to stories and how you as teacher can enhance reflection and the connectivity among stories related to teaching, health promotion, and disease prevention.

Reflection is an active, persistent, and careful consideration of any belief or supposed form of knowledge based on the evidence or grounds that support the story. Be prepared to discuss the following questions related to storytelling and reflection based upon a short lecture.

- What is storytelling, and what is reflection?
- What are the goals of storytelling and reflection?
- What are the key assumptions underlying storytelling and reflection?
- What are the essential elements of storytelling? Reflection?
- How might you use the techniques of storytelling and reflection in the classroom? During teamwork? In a clinical setting? Within communities?

DIRECTIONS

Conduct a short lecture focused on the following:

- What is storytelling and what is reflection?
- Goals of storytelling and reflection
- Underlying key assumptions

Then choose or have someone tell a story about an event or situation he or she has experienced.

Think about the questions listed next and be prepared to lead a discussion based on the story or to ask a participant to share a story to be used for discussion. Identify and discuss information related to the following questions:

- What have you learned about storytelling and reflection as learning tools?
- What are the essential elements of storytelling and reflective learning?
- How might you use the techniques of storytelling and reflection in your classroom? In the clinical setting? In the community?
- How do you assess the learning from reflection?
- What are the pros and cons of using storytelling and reflection in learning in low-resource countries?

LEARNING ACTIVITY 4.2
CRITICAL THINKING

Everyone thinks; it is human nature to do so. If left to itself, however, much of our thinking becomes biased, distorted, uninformed, or prejudiced. *Critical thinking* is a mode of thinking that shows awareness; reflection; and an understanding of one's place in the world in relation to situations, people, subjects, and other topics. In today's world, critical thinking is necessary for a person to be a fully functioning adult as well as a safe health care worker. To develop critical thinking abilities, one's educational preparation must include opportunities and experiences to practice these skills.

The purpose of this learning activity is to focus on the structure and use of selected critical thinking elements that are particularly relevant to the practice of health care workers. This exercise will provide an opportunity to use critical thinking skills related to a specific situation.

DIRECTIONS

1. The instructor will present a health-related situation that is appropriate and inherent to local settings.
2. Break into small groups. Read and discuss the definitions of critical thinking provided in this chapter to ensure that all students have an understanding of critical thinking and to build their knowledge base of the elements of critical thinking.
3. Discuss within your groups how to apply each of the critical thinking elements to the presented situation.
4. Define and list the issues/problems/questions inherent to the presented situation.
5. Determine whether there are assumptions evident in the presented situation. If so, describe them and discuss how one might verify that they are assumptions.
6. Describe the questions that need to be answered to diagnose the situation.
7. Consider how willing you are to listen to other members of the group.
8. Can any patterns in the situation be recognized? If so, describe them and discuss within the group. What supporting evidence is evident in the situation to support the description of patterns?
9. How do the contexts of culture, politics, economics, education, technology, ethics, and personal biases influence the issue(s) of the situation?

POSTDISCUSSION

As a group, prepare a brief report of the answers to the questions just listed. Choose one person to present your group's report to the larger class. After all the group presentations, work as a class identify the critical thinking elements used within the situation diagnosis.

REFERENCES

Bandman, E. L., & Bandman, B. (1995). *Critical thinking in nursing*. Norwalk, CT: Appleton & Lange.

Benner, P., Sutphen, M., Leonard, V., & Day, L. (2010). *Educating nurses: A call for radical transformation*. San Francisco, CA: Jossey-Bass.

Boud, D., Keogh, R., & Walker, D. (1985). *Reflection: Turning experience into learning*. London, England: Nichols Publishing.

Boyd, E. M., & Fales, A. W. (1983). Reflective learning: Key to learning from experience. *Journal of Humanistic Psychology, 23*, 99–117.

Bradshaw, M. J., & Lowenstein, A. J. (Eds.). (2011). *Innovative teaching strategies in nursing and related health professions* (5th ed.). Sudbury, MA: Jones & Bartlett.

Brightman, H. J. (2010). *Georgia State University Master Teacher Program*. Retrieved from http://www2.gsu.edu/~dschjb/wwwmbti.html

Dewey, J. (1933). *How we think: A restatement of the relation of reflective thinking to the educative process*. Boston, MA: Heath.

DeYoung, S. (2003). *Teaching strategies for nurse educators*. Upper Saddle River, NJ: Prentice Hall.

Ennis, R. H. (1985). Critical thinking and the curriculum. *National Forum: PHI Kappa Phi Journal, 65*, (1), 28–31.

Facione, P. A. (1990). *The Complete American Philosophical Association Delphi Research Report* (ERIC Doc. No.: ED 31542). Retrieved from http://www.insightassessment.com/pdf_files/DEXadobe.PDF

Facione, P. A. (2010). *Critical Thinking: What it is and why it counts*. Insight assessment. Retrieved from: http://www.insightassessment.com/pdf files/what&why2006.pdf

Felder, R. M., & Brent, R. (2003). Learning by doing. *Chemical Engineering Education, 37*(4), 282–283. Retrieved from: http://www4.ncsu.edu/unity/lockers/users/f/felder/public/Columns/Active.pdf

Lyman, F. T. (1981). "The responsive classroom discussion." In Anderson, A. S. (Ed.) *Mainstream Digest*. College Park, MD: University of Maryland, College of Education.

McKeachie, W. J., Pintrich, P., Lin, Y. G., Smith, D. A. F., & Sharma, R. (1990). *Teaching and learning in the college classroom: A review of the research literature* (2nd ed.). Ann Arbor: National Center for Research to Improve Postsecondary Teaching and Learning, University of Michigan.

Paul, R. W., & Binker, A. J. A. (1990). *Critical thinking: What every person needs to survive in a rapidly changing world*. Rohnert Park, CA: Center for Critical Thinking and Moral Critique, Sonoma State University. Retrieved from http://eric.ed.gov/ERICWebPortal/search/detailmini.jsp?_nfpb=true&_&ERICExtSearch_SearchValue_0=ED338557&ERICExtSearch_SearchType_0=no&accno=ED338557

Siegel, H. (1980, April). *Critical thinking as an educational ideal*. Paper presented at the 64th Annual Meeting of the American Educational Research Association, Boston, MA.

Silberman, M. (1996). *Active learning: 101 strategies to teach any subject*. Boston: Allyn & Bacon.

Smith, F. (1990). *To think*. New York, NY: Teachers College Press.

Watson, G., & Glaser, E. M. (1980). *Watson-Glaser critical thinking appraisal manual*. New York: Harcourt Brace.

5

Tools for Teaching

Many authors worldwide assert that we have entered the "age of information." They imply that our social, cultural, and professional lives are becoming restructured through the constant flow—some say bombardment—of information. We also know that access to information throughout regions of the world and within communities is not equal. Furthermore, the effects of both information overload and scarcity pose challenges for teachers and learners, regardless of their course of study. Teachers need to carefully choose sources of information that are appropriate for the course of study, guide students in finding and evaluating sources and types of information and knowledge, and make decisions as to the appropriate teaching learning methods for presenting course content. Every teacher should have a set of criteria for evaluating the sources of information they include in their course of study.

This chapter begins with an overview of sources of information, which is followed by several other related topics that can be gathered under the label *tools for teaching*, a phrase that refers to some of the concepts and techniques that enhance the teaching learning process and encourage students and teachers to work together to actively engage in teaching learning activities. Additional topics covered in this chapter include teaching knowledge, skills and attitudes; interviewing and observation in clinical and community sites; field trips to clinical and community sites, villages, and homes; guest speakers; and presentation technologies.

OVERVIEW OF SOURCES OF INFORMATION

As we begin our discussion of sources of information, two questions come to mind. First, what are the sources of information on which we rely in the health sciences? Second, how do we evaluate, analyze, and select relevant sources of information? Pondering these questions can help teachers focus on information and knowledge that are relevant to the domain of inquiry, the topics to be covered in a selected period of time, or the skills that need to be developed.

Information Versus Knowledge

The words *information* and *knowledge* are often used interchangeably, although there are differences in the concepts they represent and the manner in which they are used. According to the *American Heritage Dictionary* (2007), *information* implies a random collection of material that may or may not be relevant to the development of a coherent and orderly synthesis of knowledge; in contrast, *knowledge* refers to the range of what has been perceived, discovered, or learned and is usually related to a specific topic.

Ackoff (1989) suggested an interesting way to grasp the differences between information and knowledge in a useful manner. An adapted format of his "Knowledge Hierarchy" follows:

- *Data* refers to symbols, which can take many forms.
- *Information* refers to data that are processed to be useful and that provide answers to "who," "what," "where," and "when" questions.
- *Knowledge* refers to application of data and information and answers "how" questions.
- *Understanding* refers to appreciation of the "why" question.
- *Wisdom* refers to an evaluated understanding of the subject in question.

The important thing to remember is that information is bounded by its form in that it can be a document, an article, a speech, an observation, a news commentary, or any other form of communication, whereas knowledge has been assimilated and connected into a coherent body of related pieces of information involving experience and analysis, sometimes including apprenticeship, mentoring, and study (Pruzak, 2006).

Selected Sources of Information

Sources of information in the health sciences usually fall into a few categories. Most teachers think first of textbooks, research reports, and other forms of documentation that are generally stored in libraries, both traditional and virtual. There are also course outlines and curricula that have been formulated by faculty committees. In recent years, the Internet and other electronic sources have become available, although access can be a major problem, especially in rural areas. It is important to note that when access to print and electronic resources are not available, creative educators have made their own resource materials.

For the Ethiopia Public Health Training Initiative (see chapter 10, this volume, for a fuller description of the initiative), the modules and lecture notes being developed as part of the project had become a major source of information for both faculty and students. These modules and lecture notes were generally based on the 30 major health issues identified by Ethiopian professionals in the health sciences at the start of the project. See http://www.cartercenter.org/health/ephti/index.html for a list of the modules, lecture notes, and manuals. These materials show one model of building capacity for pre-service health education; terms of use are described on the website (International Public Health Training Initiative in Ethiopia: Carter Center Ethiopia Public Health Training Initiative, 2010). When students and educators do not have easy access to sources of information, they need to receive creative and repetitive reminders of how new sources of information can be utilized. In Ethiopia, the health sciences faculties of the seven universities assumed responsibility for developing the instructional manuals, modules, and lecture notes that have become major sources of information for teachers, students, and health center personnel. This example of how faculty dealt with the lack of access to sources of information reminds one that it is important for educators to maintain a proactive stance. The question to ask oneself is "What are the sources of information in my teaching learning situation, and how will all the persons involved learn to access and use the relevant sources of information?"

All communities have rich human resources, which often are untapped as sources of information. Human resources include family caregivers, village or community leaders, community health center personnel, patients and their families waiting to be seen by health care workers, and local and international experts/professionals. Too often, the in-country or local health care experts are overlooked, especially if it is possible to enlist the services of an international professional, yet it is the local health care experts who know the cultures, languages, and health care context.

The importance of the environmental context should not be overlooked. The environment is an essential part of the health care setting. Searching for information that relates to the environment is an important part of providing comprehensive health care in any community. A few examples include access to safe water, eliminating air pollution, disposal of waste, drainage of waste water, and availability of latrines.

One of the most overlooked and the largest untapped source of information for teaching learning is students (Guilbert, 2000). Students in low-resource countries know their communities and their families, most of whom have grappled with health and illness issues. Students will learn by engaging their community and family members in dialogue and, through the inquiry process, obtain information that is valued by their teachers.

Teachers, students, and/or workshop participants can use Learning Activity 5.1, "Overview of Sources of Information," which can be found at the end of this chapter, to learn more about this topic or to prepare for a session teaching this concept.

TEACHING KNOWLEDGE, SKILLS, AND ATTITUDES

In this section we focus on the interaction among knowledge acquisition, skill development, and the influence of attitudes in teaching and learning environments. Some people claim that teachers in the health sciences focus largely on the acquisition of scientific knowledge and the development of clinical skills while giving little attention to the role of attitudes, yet the reality is that knowledge, skills, and attitudes are usually intermingled and overlap in most teaching learning situations. It sometimes helps to think about the interaction among knowledge, skills and attitudes by using gerunds that describe the nouns: *thinking, doing, and being.*

Let us begin with working definitions of these three concepts—knowledge, skills, and attitudes—sometimes referred to by the acronym *KSA*:

- *Knowledge* refers to the sum or range of what has been perceived, discovered, or learned.
- *Skills* refers to abilities or expertise requiring one to use of one's body and/or mind to perform specific acts.
- *Attitude* refers to a state of mind or feeling with regard to some matter (*American Heritage College Dictionary*, 2007).

Another important distinction among these three important teaching learning concepts involves the domains they represent. Another word for *domain* is *category*. The distinction means that learning encompasses several types, and these learning types can be placed into categories, or domains, as follows:

- Knowledge belongs to the cognitive domain. It depends on cognition, that is, thinking about or identifying facts and ideas that are relevant to the main idea.
- Skills are most often identified with the psychomotor domain, because learning a skill often requires manual dexterity. However, in teaching skills the cognitive and communication domains are also necessary.
- Attitudes are in the affective domain, because they involve feelings and emotions.

Don Clark (1999/2009) created an informative Web page (http://www.nwlink.com/~Donclark/hrd/bloom.html) that cites the learning domains and provides a set of examples of each domain. Clark presents an update on Benjamin Bloom's (1956) earlier work on this topic while citing full references that can be useful for anyone wanting more information. He suggests that learning behaviors can be thought of as the goals of the training or educational process.

Teaching Knowledge

A body of knowledge is essential for every discipline. The health sciences have several related, though separate, bodies of knowledge that are used by health care workers who work in community health centers. These include, for example, a body of knowledge related to medicine, another for nursing, another for medical laboratory technology, and still another for environmental sanitation and health. Within each discipline there are specialties, each with their own body of knowledge, in addition to some overlapping bodies of knowledge that are shared among all health-related specialties.

One of the most difficult tasks for a teacher is to choose the specific concepts and facts that fit the curriculum; the specific class; the educational level of the learners; and the specific setting, such as the classroom, clinic, laboratory, community health center, or village. In addition, content needs to be adapted to the cultural beliefs and values of the learners and the community in which the health care workers practice. The importance of culture and learning was addressed in detail in chapter 3. Abbatt (1992) emphasized that one of the most important decisions a teacher makes about knowledge is to decide which facts are important, useful, and relevant (p. 88). This decision-making process is sometimes referred to as deciding "what must be known," often referring to it by its acronym, WMBK.

Finally, and foremost, we always need to remember that teaching knowledge alone does not change behavior. Teaching knowledge will most certainly involve the mental process of thinking, which is essential, but it must be considered along with any relevant skills that need to be learned, the attitudes held by the learners, and all other persons who are present in the setting where the teaching is taking place.

Teaching Skills

What is a *skill*? Put simply, a skill is the ability to complete a task, or an ability to accomplish something. Usually, a skill is thought to refer to something that requires the use of one's hands, such as applying a dressing to a wound. That type of skill is referred to as a *psychomotor skill*. However, when one thinks about the whole task of applying a dressing to a wound, it soon becomes apparent that some decisions need to be made throughout the process, and thus cognition, or thinking, is also involved; therefore, a health care worker needs to have cognitive skills to accomplish the task of applying a dressing to a wound. In addition, there is usually a communication component to the task of applying a dressing, and so communication skills also are needed for this task. It is now apparent that when teaching skills the teacher needs to include the psychomotor, cognitive, and communication domains. Whereas knowledge development is sometimes thought of requiring *thinking*, skill development requires *doing*.

It may be helpful to examine the *task analysis* process to understand the various types of skills needed for a given task. The task analysis process is often used in teaching skills. (For additional related content on teaching skill development and task analysis, see the discussion of competency-based learning in chapter 7, this volume.) When describing the process for teaching the task of "giving medicine by mouth," for example, the written instructions for students can be based on a task analysis (Abbatt, 1992, pp. 76–78).

The learning process for teaching skills development involves three steps: (a) describing the skill, (b) demonstrating the skill, and (c) practice and redemonstration of the skill.

Describing the skill is the first stage of teaching that skill. This should be done in a very direct, clear, and concise manner, making sure that all the learners are hearing and understanding the description of the purpose and process for using the skill. Abbatt (1992) suggested that a task analysis will be very helpful when the stages for using the skill are explained. Task analysis is discussed in more detail in chapter 7.

The next stage is *demonstrating the skill*. The most important part of demonstrating a skill is preparation by the teacher for performing the demonstration. Kroehnert (2000) suggested the following preparatory steps:

- Establish the level of knowledge the learners have regarding the skill
- Analyze and break it down into its component parts
- Draft a plan so that all relevant parts will be covered in the demonstration
- Prepare all training support materials
- Prepare learning objectives
- Prepare a good introduction for the demonstration

These steps are not conclusive but instead emphasize the importance that the demonstrator be fully prepared ahead of time.

Remember that the demonstration must be correct so that it can be replicated by the learners in their own settings. The demonstration must be visible for all the learners to see exactly what is being demonstrated, and all the steps need to be explained by the demonstrator (Abbatt, 1992).

Providing for adequate practice sessions is essential for skill development. In fact, practice and redemonstration are often considered part of any discussion of demonstration as a method for teaching skills. A good demonstrator will involve the students or participants. Ideally, the demonstrator will first perform the skill at normal speed, encouraging the students to be ready to give the verbal directions while the demonstrator goes through the skill again, more slowly. This involvement encourages the students to engage actively during the demonstration so that they will be more likely to ask questions for clarification and begin their own preparation to practice the skill.

Organizing practice sessions is often one of the most difficult aspects for the teacher. It may be difficult to find the space and time for all students/participants to practice. Ideally, practice and redemonstration should take up more than 50% of the time allotted to development of the skill. It is thus essential for all students to practice the skill, and all students should receive feedback on their performance. Redemonstration is often needed to guide some students in performing the skill adequately.

Teaching Attitudes

Some people might question whether attitudes can be taught. We will not enter into a discussion here about theories of teaching, or about concepts regarding the development and transfer of attitudes. Suffice it to say that attitudes are always a part of human interactions, including teaching learning contexts.

An *attitude* can be defined as "a state of mind or feeling" about something (*American Heritage College Dictionary*, 2007, p. 92). Attitudes are sometimes referred to as *feelings*. Earlier in this chapter, we noted that sometimes knowledge, skills, and attitudes are referred to, respectively, as *thinking, doing,* and *being*. Attitudes are part of human nature and part of who a person is, which means that attitudes shape one's *being*. Attitudes are shaped by our culture, family, education, religion, social standing, and where we live. They are part of the affective domain of psychological functioning.

The following are some of the important characteristics of attitudes in the teaching learning process:

- Expressed as an emotive tendency to behave in a certain way
- Exert a strong influence on changes in behavior and thinking
- Difficult to measure
- Hard to define or explain

When teachers learn to identify and understand their own attitudes they become more likely to provide teaching learning contexts in which students can express their feelings and recognize their own attitudes.

Even though attitudes are difficult to explain and to measure, they will always be present in teaching and learning situations. Abbatt (1992) suggested five general methods teachers can use when educating students about attitudes:

1. Provide information about the topic by showing how the facts are relevant to the attitude.
2. Provide examples or models, such as stories, pictures, and persons who can serve as role models. Remember the adage "A picture is worth a thousand words."
3. Provide experiences to shape attitudes, such as service learning (see our discussion of service learning in chapter 6, this volume).
4. Provide discussion to shape attitudes, such as case studies, small group discussion, or values clarification.
5. Use role playing exercises in which students act the parts of different people, and ask them to identify with the potential feelings those people might experience (see our discussion of role play in chapter 6, this volume).

Attitudes are the most important aspect of teaching knowledge, skills, and attitudes, but they also are the most difficult to change or influence.

OBSERVATION AND INTERVIEWING AS SOURCES OF INFORMATION

Most health professionals have been introduced to the teaching and learning tools referred to as *observation* and *interviewing* as part of their educational preparation to work within one of the health-related disciplines, yet many health professionals have not used these methods of obtaining information in many of the settings where they work; neither have they consistently taught their students about the wealth of relevant information they can gain by effectively using observation and interviewing in community health centers, villages and urban neighborhoods, and hospital and clinic settings. Students in all health disciplines need to learn the basic skills of observation and interviewing.

Definitions

Observation refers to the process of deliberately focusing on a particular scene while purposefully using all of one's senses to search for the meaning of all aspects of that particular context, including all activity within the setting. In medicine and nursing, observation is often referred to as *examination*, something doctors and nurses do all the time (Powers, 2009). There are two broad types of observation: (a) participant observation and (b) nonparticipant observation. *Participant observation* refers to the method by which an observer participates in the situation and covertly or overtly observes all aspects of what is happening within the setting (Becker & Geer, 1957). In *nonparticipant* observation the observer has only one role, that of observer, whereas the participant observer has two roles, that of observer and active member of the group (Lincoln & Guba, 1985). A nonparticipant observer usually attempts to stay separate from the situation being observed so as to minimize his or her influence on the setting. Baker (2006) contended that observation is a complex method because it often requires that the observer play a number of roles, and use a number of techniques, including her or his five senses, to collect data.

Interviewing refers to the process of gaining meaningful information about specific topics and/or situations that may include present constructions, reconstructions of the past, and/or future projections of the entities under study (Lincoln & Guba, 1985). The degree of structure of an interview usually falls into one of two categories: (a) structured and (b) nonstructured. *Structured interviews* usually are based on an attempt to focus on specific questions or topics; the interviewer uses an interview guide with a designated set of questions to be asked in the same order for all interviewees. In *nonstructured interviews* the interviewer may have a set of probes or conversation starters that are used in whatever order seems appropriate for the particular interviewee and situation. Nonstructured interviews are usually conducted in tandem with observation and are further discussed later in this section.

OBSERVATION AND INTERVIEWING IN HEALTH CENTERS AND CLINICAL SETTINGS

This section focuses on the use of observation and interviewing as sources of information in health centers and clinical settings. All health workers need to have a working knowledge of, and experience in using, these essential tools. The following discussion focuses on using nonparticipant observation and unstructured interviewing because the emphasis in this book is on the education of workers in the health-related disciplines.

Observation is a powerful tool in which one uses all the senses. The meaning of this statement is at the core of understanding the value of using observation in health care settings. Humans have five senses: (a) sight, (b) hearing, (c) touch, (d) smell, and (e) taste. Astute observers are constantly aware of using their eyes, ears, hands, nose, and mouth, depending on the situation. When observing, one is most often aware of seeing the entire situation and hearing all the sounds in the setting. However, smelling, touching, and tasting also should be used. Although these senses are not needed as often as seeing and hearing, they may be relevant.

Interviewing also is an essential tool, one that is often described as "a conversation with a purpose." The meaning of this statement focuses on the words *conversation* and *purpose*. An interview is a conversation in that both interviewer and interviewee converse and relate to each other, but there are specific guidelines as to how that conversation proceeds. The purpose of an interview is understood and agreed on by both interviewer and interviewee so that the interview proceeds according to guidelines dictated by the type of interview (e.g., structured or semistructured) and the location where it occurs.

Observation

A key characteristic of observation is the ability to collect "present time" data, in which one's own observations become the database upon which tacit knowledge is built; thus, an observer's database is composed of observed actions. The observer attempts to see the situation as the people who are involved experience it (Smith, 1997). It is always important to grasp the culture and the context of the situation being observed in its ongoing natural environment.

In nonparticipant observation the observer chooses a place that provides an ideal view of the designated site but where he or she will not intrude on the action. In some educational programs, the observation site is deliberately located outside of the usual health care settings, such as a public place (e.g., the village center or a park or marketplace). At one university, nursing students develop their observational skills in an art museum so that while they are viewing works of art they learn how to describe in detail what they see without making value judgments, rather than making statements about what they think is happening (Powers, 2009).

Some advantages of using nonparticipant observation include that the persons being observed are less likely to alter their behavior, it is rapid and easy to set up, and it is an economical way to collect basic information.

General steps in nonparticipant observation include the following:

- In a health care facility or village setting, check first with the person who has authority in the setting.
- Find an unobtrusive place to be within the setting.
- Use all of your senses deliberately and appropriately.

■ Record field notes that can later be written into a detailed record of your observations.

■ Triangulate the observation data with other forms of data, such as interviews and reports, as needed.

Finally, remember that becoming an unbiased observer is very complex and difficult. It requires one to be constantly aware of one's own culture, biases, personality, values, previous education, and experience, all of which may intrude on one's valiant attempts to be open and aware of the situation in its entirety. See Exhibit 5.1 for an example of the continuing process of learning to collect observation data. This is a story about an experience of one of the authors of this book while we were conducting the teaching learning workshops in Ethiopia with participants who were themselves university health sciences faculty.

EXHIBIT 5.1

A Personal Story About Observation

I shall always remember the incident when a workshop participant and I were doing an observation exercise in the labor and birth section of a community health center. When he reported on his observation data he described the worn electrical cords that health care workers were walking over in the examination room. I had not noticed the electrical cords, but I could describe in detail what the nurses were wearing and what they were doing. I was a nurse educator and he was an environmental health specialist. Our past experiences and education helped to influence what we noted when collecting observation data.

Interviewing

Unstructured interviews can also be referred to as *in-depth*, *clinical*, or *exploratory* interviews. Such interviews are concerned with the respondent's or interviewee's point of view and, as such, will allow the interviewer to enter into the guided conversation to probe for more information or clarification as the interview proceeds. The interviewer guides the interview with open-ended queries related to the topic of interest, prefacing the queries with encouragement phrases such as "Tell me about . . ." or "I want to learn about . . .," which will help expand the conversation. Instead of completely unstructured interviews, semistructured interviews may be used. For these, part of the interview is conducted by asking structured, usually written, questions. The remainder of the interview is unstructured, allowing for the interviewer to pose some questions that encourage the respondent to engage in directed conversation (see Exhibit 5.2).

Closing the interview is an important part of the interviewing process. The interviewer should always respect the previously agreed-on time limits and thank the interviewee for his or her generosity of time and information. It is recommended that one get permission to contact the interviewee again should clarification of data be needed.

<table>
<tr><td>

EXHIBIT 5.2

General Steps for Planning and Conducting an Unstructured Interview

1. Plan for the interview by preparing to be a keen listener and eager learner.
2. Select a process for choosing interviewees.
3. Choose a setting and time that are comfortable for the interviewee.
4. Ask for permission to take notes during the interview so that you may be accurate in recalling the information learned from the interviewee.
5. Make general "get acquainted" comments before asking some broad, general questions.
6. Move to more specific questions and comments.
7. Use probes such as "Tell me more . . ." or "Do I understand you to say that . . . . ?"
8. Redirect the conversation to the purpose of the interview as needed.
9. Briefly restate what you have learned so as to allow the interviewee to make corrections and to encourage trustworthiness and respect.

</td></tr>
</table>

FIELDWORK: AN ESSENTIAL LEARNING EXPERIENCE IN HEALTH-RELATED DISCIPLINES

Fieldwork is a necessary component of training in health-related disciplines. An essential attribute of field-based instruction is the combination of academic inquiry with off-campus activities that help students or workshop participants learn by doing in the natural setting (Davis, 1993). The goals of fieldwork are to extend and enhance opportunities for integration of theory and practice. Davis (1993) suggested several general strategies for including fieldwork in a course of study, which could equally apply when doing workshops:

- Make learning the primary objective of any field experience.
- Become familiar with the field setting before placing or sending students or workshop participants.
- Identify a specific set of activities to be undertaken while in the field setting.
- Develop written agreements and clarify the roles and responsibilities of the agency staff and the students or workshop participants.
- Know what the legal issues are in the particular sites, such as liability for the acts of students or workshop participants.
- Assess the knowledge and skills that supervising teachers and students or participants bring to the project.
- Ask all persons involved to keep journals related to the experience.
- Have frequent debriefing or reflection sessions.

Learning Activity 5.4, at the end of this chapter, relates to two sections in this chapter "Observation and Interviewing in Health Centers and Clinical Settings" and "Fieldwork: An Essential Learning Experience in Health-Related Disciplines." It provides an example of how to integrate learning about sources of information related to the skill development process for observation and interviewing with that of fieldwork in community and clinical settings.

USING GUEST SPEAKERS

Inviting guest speakers who have relevant expertise or experience is an excellent way to enlarge the horizons of students or workshop participants. The change in usual activity in the classroom or workshop helps to vary the format for the class sessions, thus increasing anticipation of something new or different. More important, guest speakers provide the opportunity for discussion of views or experiences that are different from those of the teaching team. Davis (2009) provided practical suggestions for preparing and hosting the speaker, preparing the students for the guest speaker's session, and for becoming a guest speaker.

Sometimes the teaching team includes guest speakers with the hope of providing an opportunity for students or workshop participants to actively engage in spirited dialogue. Unfortunately, sometimes such spirited dialogue does not always happen, either because the guest speaker is unfamiliar with the purpose and content of the course or workshop or because the students or participants do not understand their active role in the expected dialogue (Lang, 2008). Students may also become intimidated by a guest speaker whose credentials as a noted expert evoke awe rather than dialogue.

The following four recommendations focus on the preparation of the guest speakers and the students or workshop participants for participation in a class session (Lang, 2008):

1. Integrate the guest speakers into the course or workshop planning from the beginning. The role of guest speakers should be to help achieve certain course objectives instead of becoming an "add-on" activity or a "fill-in" when the teacher or facilitator cannot be present.
2. Select guest speakers whose work is directly connected to what the students/ participants have been studying so that the accompanying readings apply to the guest speaker's topic.
3. Prepare the guest speaker in advance by sharing the course outline or workshop agenda so that he or she will see how you intend for him or her to fit within the context of the course or workshop. It may be appropriate to have the students submit a few questions to be given to the guest speaker or panelists so as to provide information on the interests of the class.
4. Allow the guest speaker to help design how the session will unfold, including how he or she prefers to conduct the interaction with the participants, if and when any member of the teaching team will speak, and how the students have been prepared for the session.

Guest speakers can help build connections between the academic health-related disciplines and health centers and the local community. They can also offer glimpses into fields of study and practice that students/participants may one day enter.

An Example: Interdisciplinary Panel of Experts on Teaching, Learning, and Mentoring

An important aspect in planning for the teaching learning workshops in Ethiopia's Public Health Training Initiative (see chapter 10, this volume, for more details on the initiative) was the decision to emphasize active teaching learning strategies, leadership, and mentoring. What better way to do that than to include a panel of local experts who represent or teach in the disciplines of the participants in the workshops: nurses, public health officers, medical laboratory technicians, and environmental health specialists? Another goal was to promote communication and mentoring among junior and senior teachers in the health-related disciplines and health workers in community and hospital settings. Last, but not least, there was a desire to promote more reliance on experts in health-related fields within the country rather than on international health and education experts.

When choosing to use a representative panel of speakers for any teaching learning activity it is very important to establish criteria for the selection of the panel of speakers. For example, in Ethiopia the three criteria for the panel included (a) representation from the four health-related disciplines that staff the community health centers, (b) speaker location within driving distance of the workshop location, and (c) speaker willingness to tell his or her personal story in addition to values and beliefs about mentoring.

Planning for a panel of guest speakers can become quite time consuming. For example, with the Public Health Training Initiative in Ethiopia the four or five guest speakers needed to be contacted some time in advance of the workshop because most of them held academic and/or clinical positions. Each speaker was given the outline of the workshop sessions so he or she could see how this particular session fit into the whole course. The participants and speakers received a copy of Learning Activity 5.5, "Interdisciplinary Panel on Teaching, Learning, and Mentoring," which is located at the end of this chapter. Planning for the time allocation within this session was difficult because we needed to be prepared for time constraints on some of the panel members' travel to the location of the workshop, especially if they lived and worked in other cities. Although we allocated a brief time for each speaker to discuss a few of the suggested topics, many speakers chose to respond to all of the topics, which took more time than allocated. We learned that the participants entered into discussion more readily with a time schedule that included the following items:

- 9:00 a.m.: Brief presentations by the interdisciplinary panel
- 10:15 a.m.: Break (participants and panel members talked informally)
- 10:45 a.m.: Discussion time moderated by a member of the teaching team

Debriefing is an important part of this activity. Panel members and the teaching team will benefit from an invitation to review and evaluate the session. Panel members were invited to have lunch with the teaching team, during which they could have further discussion. Students or workshop participants also need to be encouraged to reflect on the experience in a setting where they are asked to think critically and speak openly about the session. In the Public Health Training Initiative experience there was a debriefing or reflection time built into each day. Each morning of the workshop began with review of the previous day's activities, so that between 8:30 and 9:00 a.m. the following day the participants were prepared to discuss their reflections on the value of the panel presentations and discussion, including suggestions for change.

This example of an interdisciplinary panel of experts on teaching, learning, and mentoring was set in a 2-week workshop for university health science faculty in Ethiopia. Please note that panel discussions such as this can be replicated in many other settings and with many other goals and expectations for the panelists and for the students or participants. Learning Activity 5.5 also can be adapted, given local circumstances and educational contexts.

USING INSTRUCTIONAL MEDIA AND TECHNOLOGY

Every teacher, including teachers in the village, health post, community health center, clinic, hospital, and academic setting, needs to know the appropriate use of instructional media and technology. The key word is *appropriate*, and appropriateness depends on the available technology, maintenance of the equipment, and skills of the teacher in using the selected teaching aids. The following discussion of instructional media and technology applies to both formal and informal teaching.

The use of learning technology varies widely throughout the world because of wide variety in the distribution of and access to technology across the globe. We begin this section by offering guidelines for using low-tech learning aids and progress toward higher tech learning aids in the following order: chalkboards, flipcharts, transparencies, slides, films and videos, and computers/PowerPoint. Exhibit 5.3 lists general strategies that apply to all types of instructional media. (For more detailed information on the following brief statements, see Davis, 2009, Section IX.)

Chalkboards and Flipcharts

Chalkboards are considered to be low tech because they require only a blackboard, chalk, and erasers. In addition, they are economical: The initial cost is low, and only the chalk needs to be replaced occasionally. Flipcharts, too, are low tech, simple in design and easy to learn to use. However, unlike chalkboards, which can be erased, the newsprint or butcher paper on a flipchart must be replaced after each use and thus can be considered costly in some settings.

Flipcharts consist of a large pad of paper attached to an easel (three-legged stand) or another type of stand. Flipcharts are best used with groups no larger than 40 persons. One can prepare the visual material ahead of time and can flip

---

EXHIBIT 5.3

General Strategies for Developing and Using Instructional Media

- Have a plan for using visual aids.
- Choose technology that is easily available and for which you have the needed skills.
- Always face the audience, glancing at your teaching aid only momentarily.
- Talk to your audience, not to the teaching aid (projector, screen, computer).
- Use titles and headings to structure your notes so the students or participants can easily scan the chalkboard, transparency, or screen.
- Use upper- and lowercase letters in a consistent manner so that your audience can quickly see words and or sentences.
- Always write or print legibly.
- Make the letters large enough to be seen easily from the farthest back corner of the room.
- Give enough time for copying, or make handouts available in class or in the library.

---

the sheets of paper as needed, or the sheets can be used for impromptu jottings during the teaching learning session. The flipchart is still the most effective presentation media for seminars and discussion groups (Laskowski, 1996).

Chalkboards

In many communities and countries where technological and electronic resources are limited, chalkboards continue to be a major teaching resource. The following points serve as a reminder for all of us to use chalkboards to their best advantage:

- *Structure the board work.* Use headings, uppercase letters, or underlining to indicate the major points.
- *Be selective.* Write down only key principles or ideas.
- *Erase old chalk work completely.* Do this before you begin your session.
- *Explain mistakes you made before erasing.* It is easy to make writing errors, but not as easy for students to know whether they may have missed reading or copying what was written.

Flipcharts

The following reminders will be useful when using flipcharts in seminars, workshops and discussion groups:

- Use 2- to 4-inch lettering.
- Highlight by underlining or writing with a different color.
- Use only red, green, brown, and black flipchart markers—yellow, orange, and pink are not easily seen.

- Keep eye contact with your audience when flipping pages.
- Always face your audience. Stand to the side of the easel, and use a pointer if needed.

Overhead Projectors and Transparencies

An overhead projector is a piece of equipment that projects enlarged images of written or pictorial material onto a screen or wall from a transparency placed horizontally below the projector and lighted from underneath. A transparency is a clear plastic 8½ × 11-inch sheet laid on top of the glass surface underneath the projector, which is lighted from below and projects in large format onto a wall or screen. Transparencies can be prepared ahead of time, which allows the instructor to choose either careful handwriting or to prepare the transparencies with a typewriter or computer. In addition to preprinting teaching materials for transparencies, the teacher can write directly on the transparency, using a non-permanent, washable, colored marking pen. The overhead projector facilitates an easy, low-cost interactive environment for educators.

Overhead projectors with transparencies are generally considered medium-level technology because they require the use of electricity, which makes their use unreliable in locations where the source of electricity is considered to be unstable. However, it is often the teaching aid of choice because it is generally considered to be more economical than using handouts. In such situations, students are responsible for transferring the information from the transparencies into their notebooks, which means the teacher needs to allow time for copying during the class session or make the transparencies available in the library or some other location.

A teacher's goal when using visual aids is to expand communication opportunities while responding to the varied learning styles in the classroom or audience. Selected recommendations intended to increase the quality of communication when using transparencies are listed in Exhibit 5.4.

Films and Videotapes

Films and videotapes are often included in the high-tech category because they require electronic equipment and skilled operators. Many educators have learned those skills but do not have much opportunity to use them consistently. In addition, access to the equipment needed to show the films or videos may be limited, even though the teacher may have access to the film or video that is related to the topic of discussion in the classroom. Davis (1993, 2009) has contended that preparation of the students or participants is an essential part of using these teaching aids. This preparation should include an explanation of the purpose of the film or video and its relationship to the context of the course of study, as well as a communication of what is expected of the learners in regard to viewing and reflecting on the film or videotape.

EXHIBIT 5.4

Recommendations for Making and Using Transparencies

- Limit the number of transparencies used in a teaching learning session—10 to 20 per 50-minute session is recommended.
- Limit text to one concept per transparency with no more than 20 to 50 words.
- When hand-writing or printing, make letters about 1 inch high for distance of 32 feet), and use 0.4-inch high letters in a small room.
- When typing, use sans serif (without tags above or below the line; e.g., Arial) fonts of 24- to 48-point size.
- Allow adequate white space between words and between sentences so as to provide enough contrast for better visibility.
- Print in upper- and lowercase letters for better visualization of words and phrases.
- Use color and graphics to highlight important points, limiting colors to black, blue, red, and green, because they produce better visibility from a distance.
- When copying a book page, enlarge it on a copier before projecting the page.
- Focus the projector before the class begins; know how to operate the equipment and adjust the distance of the projector from the screen.
- Have an extra bulb available in the classroom, and know how to change the bulb.
- Stand to the side of the projector and make sure not to block the screen from anyone's line of sight.
- Always look at the people, not at the screen or the projector.
- Turn off the projector or place opaque paper on the projector when not referring to the transparency.

(See Davis, 1993, for more detailed recommendations.)

The following list of suggested key points in using films and videotapes can serve as a guide:

- Make sure the equipment and the film or videotape are available at the time it is needed.
- Practice operating the equipment.
- Use videos/films only if they fit the objectives of the class session.
- Avoid using videos/films to occupy students' time when you cannot be there.
- Observe the students as they watch the video/film.
- Interrupt the video/film to make a point or ask questions that might enhance learning.
- Conduct a follow-up activity, such as reflection.

Computers/PowerPoint

Computers have become more common in educational contexts in recent years. Throughout the world, even in countries where educational environments have not supported electronic teaching aids because of the cost and lack of technical support, there has been rapid expansion of laptop computers and PowerPoint presentations within universities and other urban settings, such as health centers. With the advent of more powerful batteries, laptop and notebook computers have become useful for teaching in some rural and village settings.

PowerPoint is a Microsoft product widely used for presentations. It was originally designed for use in the world of business but is now commonplace in educational settings as well (Jones, 2003). Appropriate use of PowerPoint can greatly enhance both the teaching and learning experience for teachers and students. Teachers gain encouragement and support for structuring their presentation in an organized and professional manner. For students with various learning styles, the ability to mix media can make presentations more stimulating.

> Wuorio (2008) presented ways to make your PowerPoint presentation look brilliant, not brainless. One of his compelling suggestions is to remember that you are using PowerPoint to create slides that support a spoken presentation. Therefore, keep it simple and select carefully the content that needs to be visual. Remember that a diagram, a photograph, or a three-dimensional drawing, rather than printed words, may add more understanding to your spoken words.

> Computer technology has many advantages: It permits one to provide illustrations or in-depth descriptions, treat context in a different way using multiple media, and simulate dangerous or costly laboratory experiments.

The following list of suggestions provides a summary of ways to improve PowerPoint presentations:

- Avoid using high-tech learning aids to serve low-end instructional needs.
- Use standard fonts, such Arial or Times New Roman.
- Use different-size fonts for the title, main points, and secondary points.
- Use graphs or diagrams instead of only outlines, words, and charts.
- Avoid using color for decoration.
- Use transitions and animations rarely and judiciously.
- Choose a high contrast between the background and printed words—preferably a dark background and light printed words.
- Edit the slides for spelling, grammar, and repeated words.

For a summary and demonstration of the key points in preparing a PowerPoint presentation, see http://www.iasted.org/conferences/formatting/Presentations-Tips.ppt.

A final word: Always match the instructional audience with appropriate technology!

LEARNING ACTIVITY 5.1

OVERVIEW OF SOURCES OF INFORMATION

Many authors worldwide assert that we have entered the "age of information." They imply that our social, cultural, and professional lives are becoming restructured through the constant flow—some say bombardment—of information. We also know that access to information throughout regions of the world and within communities is not equal. Furthermore, the effects of both information overload and scarcity pose challenges for teachers and learners, regardless of their course of study. Teachers need to constantly evaluate the sources of information they need and should understand the criteria by which the sources should be evaluated.

DISCUSS DIFFERENCES BETWEEN INFORMATION AND KNOWLEDGE

We will be discussing the following sources of information in the next few sessions. For each resource listed, write a brief statement about how you can use it. What criteria would you use to evaluate each source of information?

- Community health centers
- Family caregivers
- Local, regional, and international experts/professionals
- Libraries
- Modules and lecture notes
- The Internet and other electronic sources
- Community leaders
- The environment
- Legends or traditional folklore
- Students

IN-CLASS EXERCISE

Each discipline group will meet to complete the following tasks:

- Select three potential sources of information
- Choose criteria for evaluating each source of information
- Discuss any relevant issues and/or barriers

When your group returns to the main session, be prepared to give a 5-minute presentation to the whole class.

   Note: This in-class exercise can be designed for any type of small group designations. This learning activity was designed for an interdisciplinary workshop, and thus the small group work was done in discipline groups.

LEARNING ACTIVITY 5.2

TEACHING KNOWLEDGE, SKILLS, AND ATTITUDES

PURPOSE

The purpose of this session is to examine the interrelationships among knowledge acquisition, skill development, and the influence of attitudes in teaching and learning environments, and to consider other sources of information about the topic. Teachers in the health sciences generally focus on scientific knowledge or clinical skills that students need to learn, giving little attention to the role of attitudes in the learning process. In addition, there are usually overlap and interaction of knowledge, skills, and attitudes in any teaching learning situation. Sometimes it is easier to think about this interaction of knowledge, skills and attitudes by using verbs that describe the nouns: *thinking, doing, and being.*

QUESTIONS

1. How would you define knowledge? Skills? Attitudes?
2. Describe how thinking, doing, and being have influenced each other in a recent situation you experienced with students.
3. How do the attitudes of the teacher influence the learning process for and with students?
4. How does culture affect the interplay of knowledge, skills, and attitudes in the learning process?
5. What other sources of information might you consider for learning and teaching about the advisability of using food-based oral rehydration therapy (see pp. 87–90)?

CLASS PREPARATION

1. Read the document "Food-Based Oral Rehydration Therapy" (food-based ORT, or FBORT), written by Dr. Dennis Carlson to several Ethiopian colleagues urging them to consider the importance of teaching about FBORT, which is presented on pp. 87–90.
2. Read this research article related to the topic:

   ■ Kassaye, M., Larson, C., & Carlson, D. (1994). A randomized community trial of prepackaged vs. homemade oral rehydration therapies. *Archives of Pediatric and Adolescent Medicine, 148,* 1288–1292.
3. Read Chapters 7 through 9 (pp. 65–96) of this book:

   ■ Abbatt, F. R. (1992). *Teaching for better learning* (2nd ed.). Geneva, Switzerland: World Health Organization.

IN-CLASS SESSION

After a brief presentation on the concepts related to teaching knowledge, skills, and attitudes, the class will divide into groups to identify the knowledge, skills, and attitudes within the Carlson document. This will be followed by a group discussion about the interaction of thinking, doing, and being in teaching FBORT and suggestions for other sources of information about FBORT.

FOOD-BASED ORAL REHYDRATION THERAPY

Introduction

The purpose of Food-based Oral Rehydration Therapy (FBORT) is for management of diarrhea and dehydration that is culturally congruent with traditional health care practices. It has demonstrated its effective use and sustainability over time. The following information includes comparison data on the use of food-based ORT with Glucose Oral Rehydration Solution (GORS), research outcomes, a recipe for FBORT, and teaching learning strategies.

Research Outcomes

Dr. Mesfin Kassaye and Dr. Befekadu Teferedegn in collaboration with Dr. Dennis Carlson and Dr. Charles Larson conducted extensive research studies on the use of GORS and FBORT in Ethiopia. Community-based randomized comparative studies were done as part of master's degree prospective research and published in international journals (Kassaye, Larson, & Carlson, 1994; Teferedegn, Larson, & Carlson, 1993).

Rationale for Using FBORT Rather Than GORS packets

There are several reasons why it is so very important to teach students in Ethiopia to understand FBORT. Since diarrhea and dehydration are still among the most common causes of death in Ethiopia, the proper use of FBORT could save millions of deaths over time in rural Ethiopia if widely used. Therefore, the following points are significant.

1. **It is impossible to get enough GORS packets into every home in Ethiopia.** Each child under five years has an average of five episodes of diarrhea a year. If there is a population of 80 million people (2010 estimate) and 20% of them are less than five years of age, that is sixteen million children in Ethiopia. When using ORS therapy that means 16 million children × 5 episodes per year × 1–2 packets per episode which equals 80 to 160 million packets per year would be needed. At a maximum, Ethiopia produces or imports 5 to 10 million packets per year. We know that the clinics and health posts are often out of ORS packets and even the logistics for delivering the available 80 million packets per year is very difficult.

2. **It is far better for the mother or other caregiver to treat the child at the home before dehydration begins and before taking the child to the health facility.** All homes have cereal flour, salt and water, so FBORT is universally available in every home in Ethiopia. Therefore, treatment for diarrhea and dehydration can begin immediately when the signs of symptoms begin. It is the dehydration that kills the child.

Learning Activity 5.2   Teaching Knowledge, Skills, and Attitudes (*Continued*)

3. **FBORT is superior to GORS packets in every way.** Studies in Ethiopia and other countries have shown that:

   a. Volume and number of bowel movements decreases sooner with FBORT than with GORS. The reason is that glucose draws fluid from the gut wall and increases diarrhea. The larger breakdown of nucleo-peptides from food slows down the excretory effect. In some parts of Ethiopia, mothers call GORS packets "Epsom Salts" because it acts to *increase* diarrhea.

   b. Children using FBORT start to gain weight faster than with GORS. The FBORT is both treatment and food. This phenomenon was found both in the research of Dr. Mesfin Kassaye and Dr. Befekadu Teferedegn.

   c. Mothers are more accepting and desirous of using FBORT than the GORS packets. The assumption is that they were more familiar with preparation of the Attimit, Gunfoo, and other porridges. In addition, there is no cost for FBORT.

4. **FBORT is more culturally appropriate and economically sustainable.** Traditionally, Ethiopians have used porridge, Attimit and Gunfoo for a long time after childbirth, injury or surgery. However, they have not used these foods very often for diarrhea until recently. However, if they learn of the usefulness of FBORT as a treatment for diarrhea, they will more likely continue because it is a modification of traditional health care. A follow-up study was done by Yifatna Timuya three years after the famine in 1984–86, when 50,000 mothers were taught to make FBORT. Three years later it was found that more than 60% of the mothers had used FBORT in the last two weeks when their children had diarrhea.

Resistance Among Health Professionals

It has been noted that despite the research results, many health professionals continue to resist the use of FBORT in preference to use of GORS packets. There are several possible explanations:

1. Some health practitioners think GORS is more "scientific." This is a natural response but not valid. FBORT has been studied in many laboratories and field trials in many countries where it has been shown that FBORT can be as reliable as the GORS packet. However, it is true that with the FBORT careful and specific training of students in the health professions, community health workers, and family caregivers is very important.

2. Health professionals think that the GORS packets are easier to use and save time for health workers and family caregivers. It is true that time in the hospital or health center is reduced with GORS packets. However, we should also time from the viewpoint of the mother and the family. Rather than needing to take the child to the health care facility, the family has the essential ingredients and will save time and money by doing FBORT at home. In addition, the child is also receiving food.

The question then arises, "How can FBORT effectively be taught to health professionals, community health workers and family caregivers?"

Teaching of FBORT

The teaching learning process should include knowledge, attitudes, and skill development. The following recipe will need to be learned by students, health center staff, and family members. In this way, communities will incorporate the thinking, feeling, and doing specifically in effective and immediate treatment at the first signs of diarrhea. The following recipe should be used for providing teaching methods and vocabulary that are appropriate to the learners. The learners must participate in actually performing the procedure of preparation of FBORT.

RECIPE

1. **Measure one liter of water into the cooking pot (equals 3 beer bottles plus 10%). First** find out what containers are used in the community such as beer bottles, cans, or larger drinking glasses. Then find out how many it takes to make one liter. Put one liter of water in the cooking pot and add about 10% more for loss through steam while boiling.
2. **Use two handfuls of flour from the household.** This may be any kind of flour, such as *tef* (local grain high in protein), barley, oats, wheat, maize, rice, bulla (cooking banana) or mashilla (millet). Every ethnic group has a preferred name for and/or type of grain that they commonly use. This amount does not need to be exact, but two handfuls are about correct.
3. **Use three fingers to pinch up salt and put it in the pot.** This may be either rock salt or traditional salt from the market, or salt purchased in the store.
4. **Bring the water, cereal, and salt to a gentle boil.** Continue a slow boil for some time. The cooked gruel should be thin enough to pour and drink.
5. **Let the FBORT cool.** It is then ready to use.
6. **Feed the FBORT to the infant or child by spoon, cup, or glass.** Replace the amount of fluid that the child had defecated. Give additional FBORT every time the child has a stool and as much as the child will eat or drink. Please note that sugar is not necessary. Most children enjoy FBORT without any sugar.
7. **Make a new batch of FBORT at least one time per day.**
8. **Continue for 3 to 5 days or until the diarrhea stops.**

Conclusion

FBORT needs to be demonstrated and re-demonstrated with faculty, students, health facility staff, traditional birth attendants, community health workers, and family caregivers. Everyone should taste the FBORT so they know it tastes good and can actually practice preparation of the FBORT porridge. Sugar does not need to be added. In many countryside communities, sugar is rare and expensive. The sodium in the salt plus the cereal breakdown products does the work.

Learning Activity 5.2   Teaching Knowledge, Skills, and Attitudes *(Continued)*

By strengthening the teaching of FBORT, you will achieve the following:

1. Save thousands of children's lives.
2. Integrate economically and culturally sustainable health care practice.
3. Use an outstanding example of teaching health behavior change that is based on sound international Ethiopian research which has been confirmed in Ethiopia. It is both a technologically and culturally sustainable health behavior.

Written by Dr. Dennis Carlson and modified with minor changes by Dr. Fran Wenger and Dr. Joyce Murray for use in the Ethiopia Public Health Training Initiative's Teaching-Learning Workshops.

OBSERVATION AND INTERVIEWING AS SOURCES OF INFORMATION IN COMMUNITY HEALTH CENTERS AND HOSPITALS

SETTING AND RATIONALE

Community health centers are the target settings for much of the community health work in most countries. In many low-resource countries, the personnel who staff these centers include public health officers, nurses, laboratory technicians, and environmentalists. The community health centers should be located where all persons in all rural and urban settings have easy access. When we promote the concept of partnering with communities, then we as health care workers are obligated to find ways in which the community health centers and the surrounding communities they serve become sources of information and reciprocal learning for health care workers and community residents. Therefore, the teaching learning strategies of observation and interviewing become essential for all of us. The same principles and techniques for observation and interviewing are also applicable in hospital settings.

CLASSWORK

1. Read pp. 169–181 on interviewing and observation in the following book:

   Lincoln, Y. S., & Guba, E. G. (1985). *Naturalistic inquiry*. Beverly Hills, CA: Sage.

   Although you will see the authors referring to using these methods in research projects, the principles are the same when using observation and interviewing for clinical and community projects and information gathering.

2. Review the document "Comparing Interviewing With Participant Observation," http://hcc.cc.gatech.edu/documents/163_Grinter_7.pdf

3. Reflect on the following questions:

   ▪ How does one decide when and how to move from informal to formal observation?
   ▪ What are the steps in interviewing?
   ▪ What are the steps in observation?
   ▪ How might you use planned observation and interviewing in your professional field?
   ▪ What kinds of information might you expect to learn from observing and interviewing in a community health center and the surrounding community?
   ▪ What are the basic skills one must develop in order to effectively use observation and interviewing?

OBSERVATION–INTERVIEW EXERCISE IN HEALTH CARE SETTINGS

We have planned for you to go in small groups to visit a health care setting, which will be in a hospital or a community health center. While there, each person will use the field trip observation and interview guide presented in Learning Activity 5.4.

Learning Activity 5.3 Observation and Interviewing as Sources of Information in Community Health Centers and Hospitals (*Continued*)

Please review the guide before the class session and make personal notes regarding how you want to use it during the field trip. It is also recommended that you bring a copy of the guide with you.

REFLECTION QUESTIONS IN PREPARATION FOR THE FIELD TRIP

- What experiences do your students have in the community health centers, such as goals or objectives?
- How are the students' classroom and community experiences connected?

LEARNING ACTIVITY 5.4

FIELD TRIP TO HEALTH CENTER OR HOSPITAL FOR OBSERVATION
AND INTERVIEW ASSIGNMENT

SETTING AND RATIONALE

Health centers and hospitals are the usual places for students in the health science disciplines to gain experience by learning how health centers and hospital service units function as an important part of the public health system. In addition, teachers help their students observe how the health center team members work together to provide health services for the people in the surrounding area. At the same time, public health practice requires that health professionals constantly search for ways to engage the people in promoting health and preventing disease, thus improving the quality of life of the community.

Skills in observation and interviewing are essential for professionals in all health care settings; however, in community settings these skills are indispensable, because professionals work with the people in community settings where we enter as guests. We learn from the people we serve about their needs while offering our professional expertise as appropriate. By using interview and observation skills we learn to understand their cultural beliefs, values, and practices so that together we can blend our knowledge, skills, and attitudes about health in ways that are beneficial in promoting the health of the community.

ACTION PLAN

Read the "Observation, Interview, and Debriefing Guide for Health Center and Hospital Settings" (presented next) in preparation for the field trip. Note the three sections entitled "Observation Time," "Interview Time," and "Debriefing Time." Students will divide into two or three groups to go to a health center or hospital and follow the directions for the activity during the observation time and the interview time as listed in this Learning Activity.

OBSERVATION, INTERVIEW, AND DEBRIEFING GUIDE
FOR HEALTH CENTER AND HOSPITAL SETTINGS

Participants will travel in small groups to visit a community health center or section of the hospital for the purpose of teaching learning field experience in observation and interviewing. **When possible, each participant will focus his or her observations and interview (optional) on the roles and functions of his or her own discipline,** for example, nurse, medical laboratory technician, environmental health specialist, or public health officer. Participants whose disciplines are not represented at the health center or hospital may focus their observations on another discipline or on patients and their families.

After a brief introduction to the health center or hospital ward, choose the setting you want to observe. You may choose to do some interviews, too. Plan for about 20 to 30 minutes of observation time. In addition to using your observation skills, you may also interview patients or personnel.

Learning Activity 5.4   Field Trip to Health Center or Hospital for Observation and Interview Assignment (*Continued*)

As soon as possible after the observation and interview time, plan to spend about 30 minutes making a record of your work. Make brief field notes while you are in the setting, recording what you observed and heard in both the observation time and the interview time. Read over your notes several times, then write a full report, recalling as much detail as you can. Record your thoughts and feelings, too, but keep that separate from the record of what you saw and heard. It is important to separate these two sources of data so that what you saw and heard is as objective as is possible, and your thoughts plus feelings become your personal reflections on what you saw and heard.

OBSERVATION TIME (FOCUSING ON THE ROLES AND FUNCTIONS OF YOUR OWN DISCIPLINE)

1. Briefly describe the setting that you are observing.
2. What are the elements in the setting that are of importance to your field of work?
3. What are the missing elements that you think are essential?
4. What do you see that the people are really doing in the setting you are observing?
5. How does what you see, hear, feel, taste, and smell relate to the health of the people and your professional health science discipline?

INTERVIEW TIME (OPTIONAL)

1. Briefly describe the interview setting.
2. What are the general characteristics of the person—gender, general age, clinic or hospital role?

SUGGESTED QUESTIONS TO ASK

1. What are the best things about working in this place? (When interviewing a patient, ask "What are the things you like about coming here for health care?")
2. What would you like to see changed?
3. What are some of the biggest health concerns in this health center (or hospital)?

DEBRIEFING TIME

The purpose of the debriefing time is for you to reflect on what you observed and persons with whom you talked, organizing your reflections around some key ideas or questions. This time is designed for us to also hear other participants' points of view, especially noting how one's professional discipline of study and practice influence what we observe.

Use the following questions to stimulate and focus your preparation for our discussion. In preparation for the debriefing time, choose one of the questions in the following list to organize your thoughts on the basis of data from the observation and interviewing you did on the field trip:

- What are the major issues facing your discipline in the community health center or hospital setting?
- What might you do to teach your students at the university about coping with these issues and becoming appropriate change agents in these settings?
- What content, skills, and attitudes do you teach students to prepare them for working in community health centers, family homes, and other community settings?
- How do you structure students' clinical experiences so that they will continually focus on empowerment of the people in order to promote the health of families and communities?
- What is the vision for this community health center?
- What improvements could be made to improve the training site?
- How might you use observation and interviewing as sources of information in any of the courses you teach or the clinical sites you use for student practice?

LEARNING ACTIVITY 5.5

INTERDISCIPLINARY PANEL ON TEACHING, LEARNING, AND MENTORING

DESCRIPTION

An interdisciplinary panel of professionals will discuss their roles and functions as faculty/professional leaders and their personal and professional journeys toward becoming experts in their chosen disciplines. The panel will reflect the disciplines of the workshop participants, namely, public health, environmental health, nursing, and medical laboratory technology. A question-and-answer period will follow the brief presentations so that the participants and panelists can engage in discussion.

PURPOSE

The purpose of this session is to provide an opportunity for participants to learn about the experiences and stories of effective teachers and their career development. This also is an opportunity to have a dialogue with educators who are experts in their professional field as well as accomplished teachers.

PANEL PRESENTATION

Each panelist will give a 10- to 12-minute presentation based on a few of the following topics. Panelists may choose to focus their comments on one or two of the topics.

SUGGESTED TOPICS/QUESTIONS

- Give a brief description of yourself, your area of expertise, and your teaching experience.
- What led you to become a teacher?
- Describe your career development, including challenges and successes.
- Discuss your perceptions of mentoring and role modeling.
- How might experts serve as sources of information for teachers in their professional field?

DISCUSSION

Participants should be prepared to ask questions or make comments related to the topics presented by the panelists or related to this session, "Experts as Sources of Information in the Teaching Learning Process."

LEARNING ACTIVITY 5.6

USING INSTRUCTIONAL MEDIA AND TECHNOLOGY

Most teachers rely on instructional media to aid them in informal and formal teaching. The term *instructional media* covers a large range of educational technologies, from chalkboards and flipcharts [flannel boards were not discussed] PowerPoint presentations and videos. For most of us, the range of options narrows depending on the context and the availability of support services such as electricity, overhead and LCD projectors, access to computers and technician assistance, and personal skills. Given the options available in any teaching learning situation, one still needs to consider the fit of the given media resource with the desired learning outcome and the skills required to use the available teaching equipment effectively and creatively.

CLASS PREPARATION

Read the following resources in preparation for classroom discussion:

▨ Davis, B. G. (2009). *Tools for teaching* (2nd ed.). San Francisco, CA: Jossey-Bass. Part IX, "Presentation Technologies," pp. 431–457. This section presents practical ideas and suggestions for the use of chalkboards, flipcharts, transparencies and overhead projectors, slide shows, films and videotapes, and PowerPoint presentations.

Wuorio, J. (2008). *Presenting with PowerPoint: 10 dos and don'ts. http://www .microsoft.com/smallbusiness/resources/technology/business-software/powerpoint-tips .aspx#Powerpointtips*

In-Class Discussion

After a mini-lecture on general principles and suggestions for using specific media, we will discuss applications for use in classroom and community settings. Be prepared to share your experiences as a teacher and as a former student in regard to the use of instructional media.

REFERENCES

Abbatt, F. R. (1992). *Teaching for better learning: A guide for teachers of primary care* (2nd ed.). Geneva, Switzerland: World Health Organization.

Ackoff, R. A. (1989). From data to wisdom. *Journal of Applied Systems Analysis, 16,* 3–9.

American Heritage College Dictionary (4th college ed.). (2007). Boston, MA: Houghton Mifflin Harcourt.

Baker, L. M. (2006). *Observation: A complex research method.* Retrieved from http://www.thefreelibrary.com/Observation:+a+complex+research+method-a0151440811

Becker, H. S., & Geer, B. (1957). *Participation observation and interviewing: A comparison.* Retrieved from http://blogs.ubc.ca/qualresearch/files/2009/09/Becker-Geer.pdf

Bloom, B. S. (1956). *Taxonomy of educational objectives: Handbook I. The cognitive domain.* New York, NY: David McKay.

Clark, D. (2009). *Bloom's taxonomy of learning domains: Three types of learning.* Retrieved from http://www.nwlink.com/~Donclark/hrd/bloom.html (Original work created 1999)

Davis, B. G. (1993). *Tools for teaching.* San Francisco, CA: Jossey-Bass.

Davis, B. G. (2009). *Tools for teaching* (2nd ed.). San Francisco, CA: Jossey-Bass.

Guilbert, J. J. (2000). *Educational handbook for health professionals* (6th ed.). Geneva, Switzerland: World Health Organization.

International Public Health Training Initiative in Ethiopia: Carter Center Ethiopia Public Health Training Initiative. (2010). Retrieved from http://www.cartercenter.org/health/ephti/index.html

Jones, A. M. (2003). *The use and abuse of PowerPoint in teaching and learning in the life sciences: A personal overview.* Retrieved from http://www.bioscience.heacademy.ac.uk/journal/vol2/beej-2-3.pdf

Kassaye, M., Larson, C., & Carlson, D. (1994). A randomized community trial of prepackaged and homemade oral rehydration therapies. *Archives of Pediatrics & Adolescent Medicine, 148,* 1288–1292.

Kroehnert, G. (2000). *Basic training for trainers* (3rd ed.). Roseville, New South Wales, Australia: Mc Graw-Hill.

Lang, J. M. (2008). Guest speakers. *Chronicle of Higher Education.* Retrieved from http://chronicle.com/Guest-Speakers/45746

Laskowski, L. (1996). *Eleven tips for using flip charts more effectively.* Retrieved from http://www.ljlseminars.com/flipchrt.htm

Lincoln, Y. S., & Guba, E. G. (1985). *Naturalistic inquiry.* Beverly Hills, CA: Sage.

Powers, J. (2009). Looking is not seeing, listening is not hearing. *Yale Nursing Matters, 10*(1), 11–13.

Pruzak, L. (2006). The world is round. *Harvard Business Review, 84*(4), 18–20.

Smith, M. K. (1997). Participant observation and informal education. In *The encyclopedia of informal education.* Retrieved from http://www.infed.org/research/participant_observation.htm

Teferedegn, B., Larson, C. P., & Carlson, D. (1993). A community-based randomized trial of home-made oral rehydration therapies. *International Journal of Epidemiology, 22,* 917–922.

Wuorio, J. (2008). *Presenting with PowerPoint: 10 dos and don'ts.* Retrieved from http://www.microsoft.com/smallbusiness/resources/technology/business-software/powerpoint-tips.aspx#Powerpointtips

6

Interactive Group Learning: The Use of Case Studies, Role Play, Simulations, Problem-Based Learning, and Service–Learning

The preparation of health care workers involves not only imparting knowledge but also developing skills for lifelong learning and promoting positive attitudes. Interactive teaching learning strategies such as case studies, problem-based learning (PBL), role play, and simulation can encourage students to apply knowledge and reflect on their understanding of theory. Each of the strategies is distinct, yet there is overlap, and they often are used simultaneously. In the broadest sense, role play, simulation, and PBL are *types* of case studies in that they use a story or problem to situate the learner in the professional environment, albeit with a good degree of variation. In this chapter we provide information on general guidelines for the use of these interactive teaching learning strategies, followed by discussion of each as separate entities.

Case studies are designed to make students apply knowledge to a realistic scenario. Strategies such as role play and simulation promote appreciation of the responsibilities of the student's future role as a health care professional. In addition, these strategies allow the students to explore their assumptions and expectations (Sutcliffe, 2002). The work of David Kolb is discussed elsewhere in the text (see chaps. 2 and 3, this volume), but we note here that his theory of experiential learning describes four stages of learning: (a) concrete experience, (b) reflective experience, (c) abstract conceptualization, and (d) active experimentation (Kolb, 1984). Simulation and role play allow students to fully engage in all four stages. Service–Learning, described in detail later in this chapter, also offers the opportunity for the student to do an activity (concrete experience), reflect back on the activity (reflective experience), think about the theoretical concepts related to the experience (abstract conceptualization), and test the theory (active experimentation). The debriefing and reflection components of the interactive teaching learning strategies discussed in this chapter foster the development of not only knowledge and skills but also attitudes (Nestle & Tierney, 2007). PBL is unique in that in its purest form it presents a scenario that triggers learning, whereas case studies and simulation require that students draw on material previously covered (Williams, 2005). A simulation or role play can be embedded in a case study or PBL.

Case studies and simulation can be done in a group or individually, whereas role plays, PBL, and Service–Learning are group activities. When done in a group, each of these methods offers an opportunity for collaborative learning and can promote an effective learning community. Service–Learning takes place outside the traditional learning environment, whereas the other four of these strategies are classroom based. We discuss each of these strategies in more detail later in this chapter. Exhibit 6.1 gives brief examples of each of the classroom-based teaching learning strategies.

EXHIBIT 6.1

Classroom-Based Interactive Teaching Learning Strategies

Example—The Girl With the Broken Heart: Hypertrophic cardiomyopathy is a leading cause of sudden death among athletes. The following exercises are examples of interactive group learning exercises and how they could be assigned.

Case study: Have the students read about a real scenario of a young girl complaining of syncope (fainting). In a narrative case, students can be given more subjective or objective information if they explain their reasons for wanting such information.

Role play: A role play exercise can be designed for students to practice interviewing a patient or delivering bad news to a patient.

Simulation: Students are told they are to take the role of a school nurse treating a girl who comes in complaining that she feels like she is going to pass out. A simulation can have students demonstrate knowledge of heart murmurs or cardiopulmonary resuscitation.

Problem-based learning: Design a scenario in which the objectives are for students to learn about hypertrophic cardiomyopathy. A simulation could be embedded in the exercise.

GENERAL RULES

The following are general rules that apply to any of the interactive methods. Suggestions for each of the specific formats (case studies, PBL, role play, and simulation) are found in the relevant section later in this chapter.

Planning and Preparation

Substantial planning and preparation are required for these strategies. Whether using role play, simulation, case studies, or PBL, there should be clear learning objectives for the session that link to the course content. As with all learning objectives, they should be developed for the educational level of the learner. Also, if possible, students should not be involved in parallel cases. In other words, faculty should, when possible, coordinate calendars so students are not simultaneously working on cases from two different sources. Such overlays can diminish the enthusiasm and effectiveness of the case method because students can become frustrated.

The teaching scenario should be realistic and meaningful to the students. Cases can be adapted from real scenarios or from the learning objectives. The level of details will differ between formats. Whole cases can be found in textbooks and on Web sites, or they can be purchased individually or as part of as a compilation. However they are obtained, the cases should be relevant to the learner. Avoid basing clinical cases on rare or obscure health conditions.

Although these strategies can be integrated into any class, it is important to pay attention to the environment. Students will need appropriate physical space to run through the role plays or simulation. In addition, a good atmosphere can promote more open interaction and sustain discussion. For in-class group work, a physical environment that allows students to face each other as they work in groups is recommended if separate break-out rooms are unavailable.

Clear instructions to students are imperative. Whether assigning a case to work on prior to class or spontaneously developing a role play, students will need clear directions, including what their responsibilities are and, where appropriate, what the expected deliverables are. Are students to hand in written reflection or reaction papers? Are they to answer specific questions related to the case? If students are to draw on external sources, clearly define the types of sources that may be used, for example, textbooks, peer-reviewed journals, and popular media. If students are not to use supplemental materials, this should be clearly stated as well.

Debriefing

Finally, students will need an adequate plan to reflect on their activities. Such *debriefing* is essential and provides an opportunity to correct any errors, make clarifications where necessary, and summarize the learning issues. Each of the specific formats may have certain ways to debrief or summarize. Be sure to leave adequate time to reflect on the sessions.

CASE STUDY

Case study, also called case-based learning, is a teaching learning strategy that uses realistic scenarios to engage the student, focusing on specific issues and relating to theory or concepts being taught (Davis, 2001; Waterman & Stanley, 2005; Williams, 2005).

Case Study Formats

Case-based learning has been used as a teaching learning strategy for many years in the fields of business, law, and medical education. It is widely used in the preparation of health care workers. Before discussing case-based learning, let us briefly look at some other variations of the case format.

Long Cases

Waterman and Stanley (2005) offered a glossary of case formats, ranging from bullet case format to the longer, extensive cases used in business and law (see Table 6.1). The extensive, or detailed case (3–100 pages) is read prior to class and worked on by the students either alone or in groups. Then, in class, the case discussion is steered by the instructor, but the students do the bulk of the work, exploring underlying issues; discussing alternatives; and, finally, proposing solutions. Students' participation greatly affects their grade (Ellet, 2007).

Short Cases

On the opposite end of the spectrum are the shortest case formats in Waterman and Stanley's (2005) glossary: the fixed choice and bullet cases. These are as short as 2 to 3 sentences. The *fixed choice case* format is frequently used in examinations, where the case is used as the stem of a multiple-choice question. The following is an example of a fixed choice case study:

> A 24-year-old schoolteacher presents to the clinic complaining of fever, chills, and headache. He has recently traveled to a malarial area. Which of the following would be an appropriate laboratory examination?
>
> a. Thick and thin blood films
> b. Hemoglobin A1C
> c. Acid fast staining

A *bullet case* also is very short and can include word problems in math. The following is an example:

> A 19-kg boy is prescribed amoxicillin 40 mg/kg/day × 10 days. Amoxicillin is available as 400 mg/5 ml. What is a single dose?

Cases of Variable Length

Among the more commonly used case formats in the preparation of health care providers are *mini-cases, directed cases,* and *narrative cases* (Waterman & Stanley, 2005). Mini- and directed cases are discussed in this section; narrative cases are frequently used in PBL and thus are discussed in that section.

MINI-CASES. Mini-cases are short (one or two paragraphs) and very focused, and they can be used in a lecture to facilitate application of the material being taught. For example, a teacher in a pharmacology class may be giving a lecture on different classes of antibiotics. A mini-case would be inserted as a scenario into the lecture, leading students to choose the best antibiotic and thus applying content just covered in a manner consistent with their profession.

TABLE 6.1		
CASE FORMATS		
Format	**Description**	**Example**
Bullet or fixed choice	2–3 sentences; student solves problem	Math problem; multiple-choice exam question with a 2- to 3-sentence case as the stem
Mini-cases	1–2 paragraphs; students apply new knowledge	Using a case in a lecture to ground the content
Directed cases	Various lengths; followed by specific or guiding questions	Previously covered content is applied
Narrative case	Longer case; case triggers learning	Problem-based learning; no content prior to case presentation
Detailed case	Very long, 3–100 pages	Case is read prior to class; class is devoted to case

Adapted from Waterman and Stanley (2005).

DIRECTED CASES. Directed cases focus the learner. However, as with all teaching, one must begin with the end in sight: What is the purpose of using a case study? The direction the case takes will determine whether the student synthesizes concepts, analyzes a situation using critical thinking, or extracts content from the case. These functions are known as *design decisions* and are intrinsic to the case. For example, if the reason for using a case is to foster critical thinking and decision-making skills, the case could unfold as the students work through it. Students would be given information as they asked for it. They would need to decide which information was pertinent to the case, demonstrating critical thinking as the case unfolds. On the other hand, in order to synthesize concepts, the students would need to have more complete information to understand the case. Specific or directed questions could then be used to direct the learning. In the case of the "Girl With the Broken Heart" given in Exhibit 6.1, to synthesize concepts related to heart murmurs the narrative of the case would include specific information about the girl's heart murmur. Students would be presented with questions to guide their learning related to the pathophysiology of heart murmurs.

In addition to the design of the case, the content must be relevant to the experience and educational level of learners, as well as to the course content, in order for the case to hold the learner's interest (Exhibit 6.2).

ROLE PLAY

Role play is defined as "an experiential learning technique with learners acting out roles in case scenarios to provide targeted practice and feedback" (Joyner & Young, 2006, p. 225). Most students find role play to be an enjoyable and

EXHIBIT 6.2

Additional Resources for Case Studies

Epidemiology case studies from the Centers for Disease Control are available at http://www.cdc.gov/eis/casestudies/casestudies.htm and http://www2a .cdc.gov/epicasestudies/

Family Health International—Training and multimedia materials are available at http://www.fhi.org/en/RH/Training/trainmat/index.htm

Herreid, C. F. (1998). **Return to Mars: How Not to Teach a Case Study.** *Journal of College Science Teaching.* Retrieved from http://ublib.buffalo.edu/libraries/ projects/cases/teaching/mars.html

National Center for Case Study Teaching in Science: http://ublib.buffalo.edu/libraries/projects/cases/case.html

About Case Studies (Pennsylvania State University), available at http://tlt.its .psu.edu/suggestions/cases

effective activity in the classroom, particularly if the scenario is well structured; relevant to their learning; and involves "choice, decision or conflict of motives" (Davis, 2001).

To design a role play, as with any other teaching learning strategy, begin with the learning objectives. Is the role play designed for the student to demonstrate knowledge, skills, and/or attitudes? Because role play enables the student to apply knowledge and demonstrate skills, these components can be worked into the scenario. Aiming at the attitudinal domain requires incorporation of choice or conflict.

Preparing for Role Play

A meaningful role play situation can be developed from real cases or even news stories. It is imperative that the scenario reflect situations that are relevant to student learning. Rare or obscure scenarios, though memorable, may not be as rewarding for the learning process, because there is less of a chance that students will encounter similar cases in their professional lives.

Provide a briefing to the group as to the purpose of the role play. Players should have a clear understanding of the details, scenario, and roles, including any specific components or information that is important to the situation. Students who are not acting in the role play can be further engaged by giving the acting students questions to consider for the nonacting students to observe. The questions can be broadly related to the scenario, or the instructor can, for example, have the nonparticipants observing the actors' body language or other nonverbal cues. As the role play proceeds, consider stopping it at a high point, where students are engaged and participating fully. This will maintain interest and can lead to a more robust discussion (Davis, 2001).

Debriefing

Discussion and feedback in role playing are critical. In addition to solidifying knowledge, they allow for a deeper understanding of the issues portrayed, clarification and elaboration of pertinent issues, correction of any errors, and exploration of assumptions (Nestle & Tierney, 2007). Davis (2001, pp. 160–161) provided some general questions that can be used to stimulate discussion. Allow participants to first review their performance, including what went well, and then address any areas of concern. Next, ask the observers to comment. Be sure to remind observers of general rules in giving feedback, such as to begin with what went well. Once the role play performances have been reviewed, move on to the broader issues to confirm that the objectives of the role play have been met.

Consider using a structured assessment form, because it "ensures the various aspects . . . are considered, and avoids omissions in the feedback session" (Joyner & Young, 2006, p. 228). Finally, take to heart Joyner and Young's (2006) last tip: Maintain your sense of humor!

SIMULATION

Simulation is a teaching learning strategy in which students engage in activities that are made to resemble the reality of a clinical practice. Simulation can be used to teach theory and decision-making skills and to assess student competency in a safe and interactive environment that mimics the clinical setting (Jeffries, 2005; Mauro, 2009). Simulations can be seen as a type of role play in that both "provide students with some form of imaginary or real world within which to act out a given situation" (Sutcliffe, 2002). Simulation has been shown to increase student confidence and self-efficacy (Nehring, Ellis, & Lashley, 2001) and is most effective when a postsimulation debriefing allows participants to review their actions and learn from mistakes (Sutcliffe, 2002).

As with any other teaching learning activity, the simulation must be aligned with the course outcomes and, as always, begin with the end, or learning objectives, in view. Furthermore, simulation scenarios should be designed with the level of learner and the competencies desired in mind. "Students' strengths and weaknesses in the cognitive, psychomotor, and affective domains should be considered as [simulation] allows learning to occur across all domains, even in a simple scenario" (Mauro, 2009, p. 30). Simulation can be of *low fidelity*, as with role play or computer flight simulators, or *high fidelity*, with mannequins that can imitate heart sounds and breathing patterns and can be manipulated on the basis of student actions. A detailed discussion on the distinction between high- and low-fidelity simulation is beyond the scope of this chapter. More important, as Beaubien and Baker (2004) pointed out, is that "when a training program is properly designed, the level of simulation fidelity becomes somewhat less important" (p. i51).

Simulations can be single events or part of a series that builds on competencies. If students are to take part in more than one simulation, a schedule should be developed that lays out the sequencing. Objectives should be **SMART**: **S**pecific, **M**easurable (in terms of performance), **A**ppropriate (to the level of the learner, the course, and curriculum), **R**ealistic, and **T**ime bound.

Faculty Guide and Script

A faculty or instructor guide can facilitate the simulation process. Such a guide would include an overview of the simulation, including the SMART objectives, and a standardized script to allow faculty to appropriately respond to any questions and ensure consistency among groups. As with a script for a play, this script includes a list of all props needed (e.g., thermometer, electrocardiogram strips, even wigs and costumes if necessary) and staging directions to set the scene for the players. Are the students in a community health center? A surgical operating room? A nursing home that has been struck by a tornado? The various roles are defined in the script. These can be shared with students so they are clear about each student's role in the simulation. However, a test run is strongly recommended before the simulation is launched with students in the classroom (Mauro, 2009).

Debriefing

As with role play, when reviewing the simulation participants should first be encouraged to explore their perceptions of the experience. A debriefing guide facilitates reflection and provides guidance for connecting the scenario to the larger learning goals. Although some simulations allow students to view their performance through videotapes, no one debriefing method is superior as long as the debriefing allows participants to identify lessons learned and develop strategies for improvement (Beaubien & Baker, 2004). Finally, the faculty taking part in the debriefing can critique the performance. It is likely that, by the end of the student debriefing, most of the pertinent issues will have been addressed. The faculty or instructor can draw attention to the learning objectives and give a summary of the simulation (Mauro, 2009; Sutcliffe, 2002).

PROBLEM-BASED LEARNING

PBL has become widely used as a teaching learning strategy in the preparation of health care workers. It is defined as "the learning which results from the process of working towards the understanding of, or resolution of, a problem" (Barrows & Tamblyn, 1980, p. 18). The literature suggests that PBL is a widely accepted, effective educational strategy (Azer, 2009; Norman & Schmidt, 2000) that has been successfully implemented in a variety of countries and across disciplines (Antepohl & Herzig, 1999; Bhattacharya, 1998; Connolly & Seneque, 1999; Khoo, 2003; Pang, Wong, Dorcas, Lai, Lee, Lee & Mok, 2002; Vittrup & Davey, 2010; Yazigi, Nemr, & Jaoude, 2004). Numerous studies indicate that the process of learning in PBL is different than the learning process in other educational techniques, producing students who are self-directed, lifelong learners (Albanese & Mitchell, 1993; Colliver, 2000; Kelson & Distlehorst, 2000; Vernon & Blake, 1993).

Theoretical Underpinnings of Problem-Based Learning

PBL is firmly rooted in the cognitive theory of constructivism. In its original form as developed at McMaster University in Canada, PBL is a learner-centered process that has at its core a clinical problem that triggers prior knowledge and free inquiry by students. The problem, which is based on, or "situated" in, health care, activates prior knowledge in the student that is then elaborated on through small group discussion in the classroom. Three aspects of cognitive psychology—(a) activation of prior knowledge, (b) situated learning, and (c) elaboration—facilitate learning and subsequent retrieval of what was learned (Norman & Schmidt, 2000). PBL educates professionals and students who can function as team members from a strong base of knowledge that they regularly update and can apply to problems (Barrows, 2000).

Process

PBL is a unique way of using and expanding on a case study. Whereas the traditional case study is teacher driven, with content experts leading students through discussion and to the answer, in PBL students work in small groups and independently between sessions to identify and build their own knowledge (Figure 6.1).

A group of five to eight students meet with a faculty facilitator, often called a *tutor*, and begin with discussion of a problem. At the first session, the group identifies a scribe or recorder to keep track of discussions. The tutor presents the students with a problem that acts as a trigger for learning. As such, the problem serves as a starting point for the acquisition and integration of new knowledge. The problem is usually complex or messy and based on a real life scenario that serves to motivate learning. Students discuss the problem in order to define it and, in doing so, come to recognize deficiencies or areas where their collective knowledge is lacking. These deficiencies are organized into "learning issues," or topics for study, and are recorded by the scribe (Greening, 1998; Koschman Glenn & Conlee, 1997). The learning issues are then divided among the student group members and researched independently between the meeting sessions. Upon returning to the group during the next session, students report their findings on their assigned learning issues. The information students present, as well as the sources of the information, is critically analyzed by the group and tutor for both validity and usefulness.

The Iterative Process of Problem Based Learning

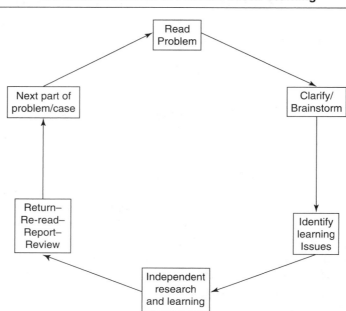

Faculty/ Instructor Role

Role of Tutor

The tutor acts as a facilitator of the group process and clinical reasoning instead of as a content expert. This role often requires a tremendous shift in power and control as the tutor transitions from the "sage on the stage to guide on the side" (King, 1993). The tutor challenges students to clearly state and elaborate on their own ideas, consider various perspectives, and critically analyze information. In addition to providing expert constraints and social support, the tutor must be aware of group dynamics and might have to intervene when problems arise.

The tutor poses probing, open-ended questions to guide the work of the group toward critical self-appraisal. The optimal group will develop a collaborative learning environment that allows universal participation, yet the tutor must be able to tolerate silence. The tutor may have to step in to promote positive interpersonal dynamics. At the same time, he or she must be able to provide direction to a floundering group and socioemotional support when group dynamics falter. It is a cognitive apprenticeship whereby tutors model expert thinking and clinical reasoning, yet tutors often need to refrain from sharing both experience and expertise, or the interactive group process will suffer.

Problem Preparation

The instructor begins by defining the objectives for the PBL. These will be linked with the objectives for the course. The objectives for the PBL will act as a touchstone as the instructor prepares the problem to depict a scenario common to the discipline. The problem should be designed to guide the students toward particular subject matter.

The problem can be developed from a real case or designed as an original case and refined to guide student learning. The case should focus on a situation that students will commonly encounter—not rare, hard-to-diagnose problems. Remember, PBL is meant to help students develop knowledge, attitudes, and skills necessary for their future job in health care. The use of rare situations can frustrate the learner.

Benefits

The PBL process fosters the development of lifelong self-directed learning skills as students recognize their need to learn and identify their own learning objectives from the given case or scenario. These student-generated objectives guide independent study (knowledge acquisition). Furthermore, situating the problem in the professional context facilitates the transfer of knowledge. In other words, when faced with problems that have similarities, students can more readily apply their knowledge rather than struggling to recall facts and theories.

Assessment and Evaluation

Assessment or evaluation in PBL is multilayered, considering both process and mastery. It is imperative to have, at the end of each session, a 10- to 15-minute informal feedback session to evaluate the effectiveness of the session in terms of content and group process. This feedback session is particularly important if the group will continue to meet.

Mastery of course content can be assessed through standard testing methods (e.g., multiple choice, short answer or essay, objective structured clinical examinations, or other competency-based assessments).

Potential Problems

PBL fosters self-directed learning skills, but successful self-directed learning requires educational resources. Students must have access to materials in order to research their learning issues. Such access is frequently an obstacle for institutions in low-resource settings. Many schools have developed hybrid styles of PBL, with lecture, simulation, and other learning sessions used as resources or complementary instructional methods (Azer, 2009; Chan, Hsu & Hong, 2008).

Preparation for the process is crucial to the success of PBL (Bhattacharya, 1998; Connolly & Seneque, 1999; Duek, 2000; Khoo, 2003; Pang et al., 2002). This preparation is especially important for students whose past education has been rooted in competitive and subject-centered methods. It is important to explain the process and benefits to the students before beginning. Group dynamics have an important role throughout the PBL process. PBL offers the additional benefit of facilitating team membership skills, which are important for health care workers, but if the group is dysfunctional then learning can be inhibited.

SERVICE–LEARNING

Service–Learning is an effective educational strategy that has been shown to enhance student learning and foster a sense of social responsibility (Eyler, Giles, Stenson, & Gray, 2003). Seifer (1998) provided the following definition of Service–Learning:

> A structured learning experience that combines community service with explicit learning objectives, preparation and reflection. Students engaged in service–learning are expected not only to provide direct community service but also to learn about the context in which the service is provided, the connection between the service and their academic coursework, and their role as citizens. (p. 274)

Service–Learning is a fine example of experiential learning. According to experiential learning theory, which is more fully discussed elsewhere in this book (e.g., chap. 2), meaningful educative experiences enhance and motivate student learning (Kolb & Fry, 1975). Service–Learning offers students the opportunity to apply relevant knowledge and skills in a real life setting. In addition, students are required to reflect on the experience. Reflection is a way for students to connect their academic study with the community service and "is widely recognized as contributing to learning that is deeper, longer-lasting, and more portable to new situations and circumstances" (Erlich, 2005). In fact, many consider the dash in *Service–Learning* to represent the reflection done by the student. Reflection (see chap. 4, this volume) helps students put knowledge and skills in context and make sense of the whole experience (Downes, Murray, & Brownsberger, 2007; Eyler & Giles, 1999). The conscious reflective activity that Dewey (1938) described allows students to "work through the attitudes and emotions which may colour their understanding, and to order and make sense of the new ideas" (Boud, Keogh, & Walker, 1985, p. 11). This is one of the unique aspects of Service–Learning as a teaching learning strategy: In addition to the knowledge and skills developed through the activity, students' attitudes can be monitored and affected.

Eyler and Giles (1999) addressed the importance of balance between service and learning. As depicted in Table 6.2, without careful design, either of the components can outweigh the other. The educational needs of students can, at times, eclipse the needs of the community with which a student is working when the *learning* of the student (i.e., service Learning) is the primary consideration. Alternatively, the needs of the community, especially when they

TABLE 6.2	
BALANCING SERVICE AND LEARNING	
service learning	The service and learning are separate, not integrated
service Learning	Student learning is the priority, with the service a secondary concern
Service learning	The service provided is paramount; learning is secondary
Service–Learning	Service and learning are balanced and explicitly linked through reflection

Adapted from Eyler and Giles (1999).

are critical, as in cases of disaster response, can lead to an imbalance whereby the *service* of the student becomes paramount (i.e., Service learning). However, with appropriate planning and coordination, an experience can be designed that balances both the service and the learning, for the mutual benefit of all (Service–Learning).

An example of such balancing is found in the use of Service–Learning as an educational experience during a drought relief program in Ethiopia during 2003–2004 (Downes et al., 2007). Of all the possible examples we could cite, we choose this example because of the severity of the situation in which the Service–Learning occurs. The following example of Service–Learning in drought relief is discussed because it demonstrates how Service–Learning can be used in even extreme and critical situations.

Service–Learning in Drought Relief

Drought is not an uncommon event in Ethiopia; a severe case occurs roughly once a decade. Ethiopian health science students therefore must be aware of the potential risks related to drought and methods of response and mitigation. Although this content could be covered in a classroom setting, actively engaging students in a public health response to a drought offers a unique opportunity to provide clinical skill preparation while also meeting the emergency public health needs of the rural populations hardest hit by the drought at the time. After careful planning among the universities and government health officials involved in the Ethiopia Public Health Training Initiative (EPHTI; see chap. 10, this volume), a Service–Learning intervention was successfully planned and executed in Ethiopia during the 2004–2005 drought precisely because it placed emphasis on balancing the services provided for the community with the learning of the students.

Before the EPHTI Drought Response Project, Ethiopian health science students would learn clinical skills through an assigned community attachment in a rural location, where activities performed were based on faculty-identified learning needs (service Learning). It is clear that the extreme demands of a drought could have resulted in Service learning, in which the critical needs of the population dictated all activities. Students could have volunteered, and their participation would have been appreciated and had a positive impact on the community. However, by carefully structuring learning activities around the community's needs, linking these needs with course objectives, and outlining the student lessons, the EPHTI Drought Response Project resulted in a balanced Service–Learning experience. The success of this particular drought response was made possible through student participation and demonstrates how, even under less-than-optimal conditions, the students' learning needs can be balanced with the community's needs through a well-designed Service–Learning experience. The extreme needs of this population in crisis could have precluded any effort to balance the service and learning.

Principles of Service–Learning

As described earlier in this chapter, a successful Service–Learning experience requires advance planning. How is this accomplished? In his list of "Principles of Good Practice for Service Learning Pedagogy," Howard (2001) pointed out that academic rigor should not be compromised (Principle 2) for a Service–Learning project and that academic credit should be given for learning, not service (Principle 1) (Figure 6.2). This balance requires assessment of student learning rather than just participation. Therefore, learning objectives should be clearly stated, with measurable outcomes (Principle 3), and the location of the service should meet established criteria (Principle 4). The expectations for the students should be clearly stated, and the service activities should "promote critical reflection, analysis, and application of service experiences [to] enable learning" (p. 17) and promote civic engagement (Principles 5 and 6). The use of group assignments facilitates civic engagement as opposed to the private learning of individual assignments (Principle 10).

As stated earlier, one of the benefits of experiential learning is that it is "portable." Traditionally, the classroom is very much teacher centered, with the student being in the passive role. Service–Learning, however, requires the student to be an active participant in his or her own learning. Therefore, the experience is designed to be student centered and then brought back to the classroom, allowing the student to apply the experience to the course content and vice versa (Howard, 2001, Principle 7). This type of experience may require transition by the instructor role from one of "knowledge transmitter" to facilitator (Howard, 2001, Principle 8). Such a transfer necessitates a shift of control and requires flexibility on the parts of all involved (Howard, 2001, Principle 9).

Use of Reflection in Service–Learning

One cannot assume that learning has occurred simply because the Service–Learning activity has been completed. It is imperative to link the service activity to the course through deliberate, well-structured reflection. The course objectives

FIGURE 6.2

Principles of Good Practice for Service Learning Pedagogy*

Principle 1: Academic Credit Is for Learning, Not for Service

This first principle speaks to those who puzzle over how to assess students' service in the community, or what weight to assign community involvement in f nal grades.

In traditional courses, academic credit and grades are assigned based on students' demonstration of academic learning as measured by the instructor. It is no different in service learning courses. While in traditional courses we assess students' learning from traditional course resources, e.g., textbooks, class discussions, library research, etc., in service learning courses we evaluate students' learning from traditional resources, from the community service, and from the blending of the two. So, academic credit is not awarded for doing service or for the quality of the service, but rather for the student's demonstration of academic and civic learning.

Principle 2: Do Not Compromise Academic Rigor

Since there is a widespread perception in academic circles that community service is a "soft" learning resource, there may be a temptation to compromise the academic rigor in a service learning course.

Labeling community service as a "soft" learning stimulus reflects a gross misperception. The perceived "soft" service component actually raises the learning challenge in a course. Service learning students must not only master academic material as in traditional courses, but also learn how to learn from unstructured and ill-structured community experiences and merge that learning with the learning from other course resources. Furthermore, while in traditional courses students must satisfy only academic learning objectives; in service learning courses students must satisfy both academic and civic learning objectives. All of this makes for challenging intellectual work, commensurate with rigorous academic standards.

Principle 3: Establish Learning Objectives

It is a service learning maxim that one cannot develop a quality service learning course without first setting very explicit learning objectives. This principle is foundational to Service Learning, and serves as the focus of sections four and five of this workbook.

While establishing learning objectives for students is a standard to which all courses are accountable, in fact, it is especially necessary and advantageous to establish learning objectives in service learning courses. The addition of the community as a learning context multiplies the learning possibilities. To sort out those of greatest priority, as well as to leverage the bounty of learning opportunities offered by community service experiences, deliberate planning of course academic *and* civic learning objectives is required.

*Reprinted by permission of the author. Updated from the original: Howard, J. (1993)."Community service learning in the curriculum." In J. Howard (Ed.), Praxis I: A faculty casebook on community service learning. (pp. 3-12). Ann Arbor: OCSL Press.

(Continued)

FIGURE 6.2   *(Continued)*

Principle 4: Establish Criteria for the Selection of Service-Placements

Requiring students to serve in *any* community-based organization as part of a Service Learning courses is tantamount to requiring students to read *any* book as part of a traditional course.

Faculty who are deliberate about establishing criteria for selecting community service placements will find that students are able to extract more relevant learning from their respective service experiences, and are more likely to meet course learning objectives.

We recommend four criteria for selecting service placements:

1   Circumscribe the range of acceptable service placements around the content of the course (e.g., for a course on homelessness, homeless shelters and soup kitchens are learning-appropriate placements, but serving in a hospice is not).
2   Limit specific service activities and contexts to those with the potential to meet course-relevant academic and civic learning objectives (*e.g.,* filing papers in a warehouse while of service to a school district will offer little to stimulate either academic or civic learning in a course on elementary school education).
3   Correlate the required duration of service with its role in the realization of academic and civic learning objectives (*e.g.,* one two-hour shift at a hospital will do little to contribute to academic or civic learning in a course on institutional healthcare).
4   Assign community projects that meet real needs as determined by the community.

Principle 5: Provide Educationally-Sound Learning Strategies to Harvest Community Learning and Realize Course Learning Objectives

Requiring Service Learning students to merely record their service activities and hours as their journal assignment is tantamount to requiring students in an engineering course to log their activities and hours in a lab.

Learning in any course is realized by an appropriate mix and level of learning strategies and assignments that correspond with the learning objectives for the course. Given that in service learning courses we want to utilize students' service experiences in part to achieve academic and civic course learning objectives, learning strategies must be employed that support learning from service experiences and enable its use toward meeting course learning objectives.

Learning interventions that promote critical reflection, analysis, and application of service experiences enable learning. To make certain that service does not underachieve in its role as an instrument of learning, careful thought must be given to learning activities that encourage the integration of experiential and academic learning. These activities include classroom discussions, presentations, and journals and paper assignments that support analysis of service experiences in the context of the course academic and civic learning objectives. Of course, clarity about course learning objectives is a prerequisite for identifying educationally-sound learning strategies.

FIGURE 6.2   *(Continued)*

Principle 6: Prepare Students for Learning from the Community

Most students lack experience with both extracting and making meaning from experience and in merging it with other academic and civic course learning strategies.

Therefore, even an exemplary reflection journal assignment will yield, without sufficient support, uneven responses. Faculty can provide: (1) learning supports, such as opportunities to acquire skills for accumulating the learning from the service context (*e.g.,* participant-observer skills), and/or (2) examples of how to successfully complete assignments (e.g., make past exemplary student papers and reflection journals available to current students to peruse).

Menlo (1993) identifies four competencies to accentuate student learning from the community: reflective listening, seeking feedback, acuity in observation, and mindfulness in thinking.

Principle 7: Minimize the Distinction Between the Students' Community Learning Role and Classroom Learning Role

Classrooms and communities are very different learning contexts. Each requires students to assume a different learner role. Generally, classrooms provide a high level of teacher direction, with students expected to assume mostly a passive learning role. In contrast, service communities usually provide a low level of teaching direction, with students expected to assume mostly an active learner role. Alternating between the passive learning role in the classroom and the active learning role in the community may challenge and even impede student learning. The solution is to shape the learning environments so that students assume similar learning roles in both contexts.

While one solution is to intervene so that the service community provides a high level of teaching direction, we recommend, for several reasons, modifying the traditional classroom toward one that values students as active learners. First, active learning is consistent with active civic participation that service learning seeks to foster. Second, students bring information from the community to the classroom that can be utilized on behalf of others' learning. Finally, we know from recent research in the field of cognitive science that students develop deeper understanding of course material if they have an opportunity to actively construct knowledge (Eyler & Giles, 1999).

Principle 8: Rethink the Faculty Instructional Role

If faculty encourage students' active learning in the classroom, what would be a concomitant and consistent change in one's teaching role?

Commensurate with the preceding principle's recommendation for an active student learning posture, this principle advocates that Service Learning teachers, too, rethink their roles. An instructor role that would be most compatible with an active student role shifts away from a singular reliance on transmission of knowledge and toward mixed pedagogical methods that include learning facilitation and guidance. Exclusive or even primary use of traditional instructional models, *e.g.,* a banking model (Freire, 1970), interferes with the promise of learning in Service Learning courses.

To reshape one's classroom role to capitalize on the learning bounty in Service Learning, faculty will find Howard's (1998) model of "Transforming the Classroom" helpful. This four stage model begins with the traditional

FIGURE 6.2 *(Continued)*

classroom in which students are passive, teachers are directive, and all conform to the learned rules of the classroom. In the second stage, the instructor begins to resocialize herself toward a more facilitative role; but the students, socialized for many years to be passive learners, are slow to change to a more active mode. In the third stage, with the perseverance of the instructor, the students begin to develop and acquire the skills and propensities to be active in the classroom. Frequently, during this phase, faculty will become concerned that the learning is not as rich and rigorous as when they are using the more popular lecture format, and may regress to a more directive posture. Over time homeostatis is established, and the instructor and the students achieve an environment in which mixed pedagogical methods lead to students who are active learners, instructors fluent in multiple teaching methods, and strong academic and civic learning outcomes.

Principle 9: Be Prepared for Variation in, and Some Loss of Control with, Student Learning Outcomes

For those faculty who value homogeneity in student learning outcomes, as well as control of the learning environment, Service Learning may not be a good fit.

In college courses, learning strategies largely determine student outcomes, and this is true in Service Learning courses, too. However, in traditional courses, the learning strategies (i.e., lectures, labs, and readings) are constant for all enrolled students and under the watchful eye of the faculty member. In Service Learning courses, given variability in service experiences and their influential role in student learning, one can anticipate greater heterogeneity in student learning outcomes and compromises to faculty control. Even when Service Learning students are exposed to the same presentations and the same readings, instructors can expect that classroom discussions will be less predictable and the content of student papers/projects less homogeneous than in courses without a service assignment. As an instructor, are you prepared for greater heterogeneity in student learning outcomes and some degree of loss in control over student learning stimuli?

Principle 10: Maximize the Community Responsibility Orientation of the Course

This principle is for those who think that civic learning can only spring from the community service component of a course.

One of the necessary conditions of a Service Learning course is purposeful civic learning. Designing classroom norms and learning strategies that not only enhance academic learning but also encourage civic learning are essential to purposeful civic learning. While most traditional courses are organized for private learning that advances the individual student, Service Learning instructors should consider employing learning strategies that will complement and reinforce the civic lessons from the community experience. For example, efforts to convert from individual to group assignments and from instructor only to instructor and student review of student assignments, modifies the teaching learning process to be consistent with the civic orientation of Service Learning.

will guide the selection of the most appropriate types of reflection. Instructors must also consider how the Service–Learning fits into the course and curriculum. Feedback on reflection is imperative, so instructors must determine the timing and frequency of the reflection. Although frequent reflection may optimize the links between experience and coursework, it might be harder to give timely feedback to frequent reflections in a large class. Although students are graded on academic performance, not hours of service, the grading for Service–Learning must reflect the time required to complete the activity and the necessary reflection, and must also fit into the course grade. Students will inevitably get a mixed message if their grade reflects their performance on examinations rather than their efforts in Service–Learning (for more discussion of reflection, see chap. 2, this volume).

Community Engagement Through Service–Learning

In a broader sense, Service–Learning can also be seen as a strategy for community engagement. In discussing university and community partnerships, Rich, Engle, and Hartfield-Mendez (2010) differentiated levels of engagement. Volunteerism, at one end of the spectrum, can be seen as service *for* learning. It is an introduction, with limited exposure, to issues or communities, and it occurs over short periods of time. A more engaged model connects the classroom to the community by designing the activity as part of the course. Such engagement is Service–Learning because, in addition to offering credit for the activity, the experience is linked to the required course learning through application and reflection. However, limiting the activity to one course would be seen as an intermediate level of community engagement. Deeper engagement requires structured academic programs and a sustained relationship with partners. This level of engagement goes beyond individual student learning and is measured in terms of community outcomes as well. Deeper engagement makes transformation possible through truly collaborative processes.

Service–Learning is a rich, well-established pedagogical approach; however, it is vastly different from other teaching learning strategies, such as lecture. Service–Learning is experiential and necessitates a shift in control away from the teacher to the learner and, to some extent, the community partner, who should have substantial input into the planning and design of the activities.

HELPFUL LINK

Campus Compact is a national coalition of more than 1,100 college and university presidents—representing some 6 million students—dedicated to promoting community service, civic engagement, and Service–Learning in higher education. See http://www.compact.org/.

DEVELOPING A CASE FOR CASE STUDIES, PROBLEM-BASED LEARNING, SIMULATION, OR ROLE PLAY

DIRECTIONS

Use the following outline as a guide to develop a scenario.

1. **For which course is this scenario intended? Is it part of a series?**
2. **Overall concepts and primary learning objectives or outcomes**
   a. **Overall concepts:** What is the main subject being addressed? This section is intended to prepare faculty/tutors to assist the students. Include references so the tutor might refresh his or her knowledge of the subject, if necessary.
   b. **Primary learning objectives:** State the objectives/outcomes for this scenario. They should be **SMART**: **S**pecific, **M**easurable, **A**ppropriate (to the educational level of the learner, course, and curriculum), **R**ealistic, and **T**ime bound.
3. **What other topics or enabling objectives are goals of the course?** This information can be shared with the students prior to the case study or simulation. What will facilitate learning or assist the student with the case? Be specific and include things the student could review beforehand, such as knowledge and skills related to the subject matter that has already been covered (e.g., anatomy, physiology, specific skills). Such prior sharing of information would not apply to problem-based learning scenarios, for which the student would need to arrive "cold."
4. **Rationale:** How does this topic fit within the bigger picture of the student's education? Why is this particular topic important? The answers may involve local demographics, including data on morbidity/mortality related to the subject.
5. **Linked concepts:** Has related content been previously covered in this or other courses?
6. **Professional or core competencies:** Which of the established professional or core competencies does this scenario address?

LEARNING ACTIVITY 6.2

SERVICE–LEARNING

Overview: What is Service–Learning?

Service–Learning is a method by which students learn and apply knowledge while addressing real problems in the communities being served. Seifer (1998) defined it as follows:

> A structured learning experience that combines community service with explicit learning objectives, preparation and reflection. Students engaged in service–learning are expected not only to provide direct community service but also learn about the context in which the service is provided, the connection between the service and their academic coursework, and their role as citizens. (p. 274)

In Service–Learning there is a clear link between the learning objectives and the service experience that is based on the assets and needs of the community. The experience is integrated into the curriculum, is developed and coordinated with the community, and provides a structured time for student reflection.

DIRECTIONS

1. Read the following article:
   Wondimikun, Y., Feleke, A., & Tafete, M. (2005). Successful coupling of community attachment of health science students with relief work for drought victims. *Education for Health, 18,* 179–193. Retrieved from http://www.educationfor-health.net/EfHArticleArchive/1357-6283_v18n2s7_713994314.pdf
2. Consider the following while reading the article:
   - How is community health organized at your institution?
   - How was the attachment described in the article different from the community health rotation at your institution?
   - How was the attachment evaluated?
3. Present a brief lecture and do small group work:
   (a) Differentiate between standard clinical attachments and a Service–Learning activity.
   (b) Using the attached "Developing a Service-Learning Experience," design a Service–Learning activity for your institution.

LEARNING ACTIVITY 6.3

DEVELOPING A SERVICE-LEARNING EXPERIENCE

Why is Service–Learning being incorporated into this course? Which reasons are most important? Which course objectives are linked with this activity?

What is the service that students will be performing for this course? How does it link with the objectives?

Direct: Students will work directly with community members. Examples include providing after-school tutoring, offering foot care to homeless populations, administering flu shots in a community setting, working with refugees in English-as-a-second-language program.

Non-Direct: Students work with an agency to facilitate its mission but do not provide direct services. Examples include packing meals for shut-ins, sorting medical supplies for a mission trip, developing and updating an inventory system, filing and helping with paperwork.

Indirect: Students engage in advocacy. Examples include contacting elected officials related to an issue of concern for the community being served, fundraising, collecting supplies for a women and children's shelter.

Are there readings or other assignments that link to the objectives and/or the service?

What will the students need to turn in to the instructor to receive credit? How will the course credit be awarded?

- Will all students be with the same partner?
- How much time is required for full participation?
- Is the Service–Learning activity required for class credit?

What types of reflection will you use? (Journal, oral presentation, etc.)

For more information on reflection assignments, see *http://emedia.leeward.hawaii.edu/servicelearning/reflection.htm*

Sources: The Faculty Handbook for Service Learning, University of Maryland, 1999, available from http://www.csl.umd.edu/faculty_staff/ServiceLearning.pdf; Service Learning Development Form, Volunteer Action Center, Florida International University, 2010, available from http://www2.fiu.edu/~time4chg/Library/devfrom.html; and Leeward Community College (2010). Service-Learnning Development Worksheet available from http://emedia.leeward.hawaii.edu/servicelearning/worksheet.htm

REFERENCES

Albanese, M. A., & Mitchell, S. (1993). Problem-based learning: A review of literature on its outcomes and implementation issues. *Academic Medicine, 68,* 52–81.

Antepohl, W., & Herzig, S. (1999). Problem-based learning versus lecture-based learning in a course of basic pharmacology: A controlled, randomized study. *Medical Education, 33,* 106–113.

Azer, S. (2009). What makes a great lecture? Use of lectures in a hybrid PBL curriculum. *Kaohsiung Journal of Medical Science, 25,* 109–115.

Barrows, H. (2000). Foreword. In D. H. Evensen & C. E. Hmelo-Silver (Eds.), *Problem-based learning: A research perspective on learning interactions* (pp. vii–ix). Mahwah, NJ: Erlbaum.

Barrows, H., & Tamblyn, R. M. (1980). *Problem-based learning: An approach to medical education.* New York, NY: Springer Publishing.

Beaubien, J., & Baker, D. (2004).The use of simulation for training teamwork skills in health care: How low can you go? *Quality and Safety in Health Care, 13,* i51–i56. doi:10.1136/qshc.2004.009845

Bhattacharya, N. (1998). Students' perceptions of problem-based learning at the B.P. Koirala Institute of Health Sciences, Nepal. *Medical Education, 32,* 407–410.

Boud, D., Keogh, R., & Walker, D. (1985). *Reflection: Turning experience into learning.* London, England: Kogan Page.

Chan, W., Hsu, C., & Hong, C. (2008). Innovative "Case-Based Integrated Teaching" in an undergraduate medical curriculum: development and teachers' and students' responses. *Annals, Academy of Medicine, Singapore 37, (11)* 952–956.

Colliver, J. A. (2000). Effectiveness of PBL curricula. *Medical Education, 34,* 959–960.

Connolly, C., & Seneque, M. (1999). Evaluating problem-based learning in a multilingual student population. *Medical Education, 33,* 738–744.

Davis, B. (2001). *Tools for teaching.* San Francisco, CA: Jossey-Bass.

Dewey, J. (1938). *Experience and education.* New York, NY: Macmillan.

Downes, E., Murray, J., & Brownsberger, S. (2007). The use of service–learning in drought response by universities in Ethiopia. *Nursing Outlook, 55,* 224–231.

Duek, J. (2000). Whose group is it, anyway? Equity of student discourse in problem-based learning. In D. H. Evensen & C. Hmelo (Eds.), *Problem-based learning: A research perspective on learning interactions* (pp. 75–107). Mahwah, NJ: Erlbaum.

Ehrlich, T. (2005, July). Service–learning in undergraduate education: Where is it going? *Carnegie Perspectives.* Retrieved from http://www.carnegiefoundation.org/perspectives/service-learning-undergraduate-education-where-it-going

Ellet, W. (2007). *Case study handbook: How to read, discuss, and write persuasively about cases.* Boston, MA: Harvard Business Press.

Eyler, J., & Giles, D. (1999). *Where's the learning in service–learning?* San Francisco, CA: Jossey-Bass.

Eyler, J., Giles, D. E., Stenson, C. M., & Gray, C. (2003). At a glance: What we know about the effects of service–learning on college students, faculty, institutions and communities 1993–2000. In *Introduction to Service–Learning Toolkit* (2nd ed., pp. 15–19). Providence, RI: Brown University.

Greening, T. (1998). Scaffolding for success in PBL. *Medical Education Online, 3*(4). Retrieved from http://www.med-ed-online.org/f0000012.htm

Howard, J. (2001). Principles of good practice for service-learning pedagogy. *Michigan Journal of Community Service Learning, Summer 2001,* 16–19.

Jeffries, P. (2005). A framework for designing, implementing, and evaluating simulations used as teaching strategies in nursing. *Nursing Education Perspectives, 26,* 96–103.

Joyner, B., & Young, L. (2006). Teaching medical students using role play: Twelve tips for successful role plays. *Medical Teacher, 28,* 225–229.

Kelson, A., & Distlehorst, L. (2000). Groups in problem-based learning (PBL): Essential elements in theory and practice. In D. Evensen & C. Hmelo (Eds.), *Problem-based learning: A research perspective on learning interactions* (pp. 167–184). Mahwah, NJ: Erlbaum.

Khoo, H. E. (2003). Implementation of problem-based learning in Asian medical schools and students' perceptions of their experience. *Medical Education, 37,* 401–409. doi:10.1046/j.1365-2923.2003.01489.x

King, A. (1993). From sage on the stage to guide on the side. *College Teaching, 41,* 30–35.

Kolb, D., & Fry, R. (1975). Toward an applied theory of experiential learning. In C. Cooper (Ed.), *Theories of group process.* London, England: Wiley.

Kolb, D. (1984). *Experiential learning: Experience as the source of learning and development.* Englewood Cliffs, NJ: Prentice Hall.

Koschman, T., Glenn, P., & Conlee, M. (1997). Analyzing the emergence of a learning issue in problem-based learning. *Medical Education Online, 2*(2). Retrieved from http://www.med-ed-online.net/index.php/meo/article/viewFile/4290/4481

Mauro, A. (2009). Jumping on the simulation bandwagon: Getting started. *Teaching and Learning in Nursing, 4,* 30–33.

Nehring, W. M., Ellis, W. E., & Lashley, F. R. (2001). Human patient simulators in nursing education: An overview. *Simulation & Gaming, 32,* 194–204.

Nestle, D., & Tierney, T. (2007). Role-play for medical students learning about communication: Guidelines for maximising benefits. *BMC Medical Education, 7*(3). Retrieved from: http://www.biomedcentral.com/1472-6920/7/3

Norman, G. R., & Schmidt, H. G. (2000). Effectiveness of problem-based learning curricula: Theory, practice and paper darts. *Medical Education, 34,* 721–728.

Pang, S. M., Wong, T. K., Dorcas, A., Lai, C. K., Lee, R. L., Lee, W. M., & Mok, E. S. (2002). Evaluating the use of developmental action inquiry in constructing a problem-based learning curriculum for pre-registration nursing education in Hong Kong: A student perspective. *Journal of Advanced Nursing, 40,* 230–241.

Rich, M., Engle, S., & Hartfield-Mendez, V. (2010). *Connecting campus to community: A place-based strategy for preparing engaged scholars* [PowerPoint slides]. Retrieved from https://classes.emory.edu/webapps/portal/frameset.jsp?tab=community&url=%2Fbin%2Fcommon%2Fcourse.pl%3Fcourse_id%3D_20917_1

Seifer, S. D. (1998). Service–learning: Community–campus partnerships for health professions education. *Academic Medicine, 73,* 273–277.

Sutcliffe, M. (2002, September). Simulations, games and role-play. In P. Davies (Ed.), *The handbook for economics lecturers.* Retrieved from http://www.economicsnetwork.ac.uk/handbook/games/

Vernon, D. T., & Blake, R. L. (1993). Does problem-based learning work? A meta-analysis of evaluative research. *Academic Medicine, 68,* 550–563.

Vittrup, A. & Davey, A. (2010). Problem-based learning— "Bringing everything together"— a strategy for graduate nurse programs. *Nurse Education in Practice 10,* (2) 88–95.

Waterman, M., & Stanley, E. (2005). *Case format variations.* Retrieved from http://cstl-csm.semo.edu/waterman/CBL/Caseformats.html

Williams, B. (2005). Case based learning—A review of the literature. Is there scope for this educational paradigm in prehospital education? *Emergency Medicine Journal, 22,* 577–581. doi:10.1136/emj.2004.022707

Yazigi, A., Nemr, E., & Jaoude, A. (2004). Implementation of problem-based learning in Asia: Similarities between Far East and Middle East medical schools. *Medical Education, 38,* 223. doi:10.1111/j.1365-2923.2004.01758.x

7

Teaching in a Clinical Setting

Teaching in a clinical setting can be challenging. The students' goals are to apply knowledge, develop clinical skills, and refine judgment as they transition into the professional role, and the instructor must not only help guide them toward these goals but also ensure safety and positive outcomes for the patients. In addition to these competing demands, the instructor often has little control over certain aspects of the learning environment, such as severity of patient illness; staffing; matching student and patient needs and numbers; and, invariably, time limitations.

There is a growing body of knowledge indicating that effective clinical teachers have distinct professional and personal attributes; specifically, they are competent, inspiring role models who stimulate learning through actively engaging the student. They have good interpersonal skills that foster communication and support. (Bradshaw, 2011; Masunaga & Hitchcock, 2010; Molodysky, 2006; Sutkin, Wagner, Harris, & Schiffer, 2008). However, clinical teaching does not happen in isolation. Throughout the world, clinical teaching occurs in complex and dynamic settings that influence learning (Pratt, Harris, & Collins, 2009; Wall et al., 2009). It is imperative that this context be taken into consideration when evaluating clinical teaching.

In this chapter we discuss some strategies that are effective in the clinical setting to actively engage students and enhance their interpersonal skills. Consideration will be given to the context in which learning takes place. There will be only limited discussion of educational theory and adult learning, because those topics were more fully addressed in chapter 2.

PREPARATION

Know the Curriculum

It is imperative that the clinical instructor understands where the clinical course fits into the curriculum overall and, more specifically, the expected objectives or outcomes for the clinical assignment. Students in the earlier stages of a program will need more direction and will be more dependent on the instructor's expertise (Grow, 1991/1996; Lacasse, Lee, Ghavam-Rassoul, & Batty, 2009). Some courses will have specific clinical requirements. Students may need to demonstrate proficiency of specific skills and stated competencies by logging a certain number of procedures, such as a minimum number of newborn baby examinations or specified number of lumbar punctures. It is the instructor's responsibility to be aware of these requirements and facilitate the students' opportunities for successful completion.

Know the Learner

It is important for instructors to know the educational level of students[1] in order to appropriately assign work in a clinical setting. Each student needs help in making the transition from dependent learner to self-directed learner. In addition, each new clinical rotation may begin with the students, even the most self-directed ones, needing some assistance. It may be helpful to develop specific goals for each learner. This is best done in collaboration with the learner (Irby & Wilkerson, 2008).

Know the Site

The clinical instructor should, at a minimum, visit the clinical site before the students do. Often, clinical instructors are employed part or full time at the clinical site and thus are already familiar with the site's layout, ancillary staff, and policies and procedures. For instructors who are not based at the clinical site, a formal orientation is sometimes available, and participation is highly recommended. Where that is not the case, it is the clinical instructor's responsibility to visit the clinical site before bringing students there, to become familiar with the staff, physical layout, policies and procedures, and issues related to documentation (Bradshaw, 2011).

It is important that the instructor know the site because, as mentioned earlier, learning does not happen in isolation. It is clear that the learning environment, the context in which the learning is to happen, has an impact (Dornan, Boshuizen, King, & Scherpbier, 2007; Pratt, Harris, & Collins, 2009; Roff, McAleer, & Skinner, 2005). Students must be allowed to fully engage in their learning and be supported by the entire team at the clinical setting. Pratt et al. (2009) eloquently described the merits of engagement related to student learning in the clinical setting:

> Engagement refers to a quality of activity that is challenging and worthy, but within the bounds of one's ability ... It means learners are doing authentic tasks alongside members of the community they want to join. By doing authentic work alongside co-workers, learners are deeply engaged in learning both the work and the normative ways of the

---

[1]Educational student level refers to whether a student is a beginner or more advanced in their program of study (i.e., first year or final year students). Expectations of students just beginning a program will be different than that of students who have more experience or education, and the evidence-based teaching strategies employed should take these various educational and experience levels into consideration.

community they wish to join. In this context, authentic work is work that has an impact on patient care and is perceived by the students as relevant to their training. They are learning a body of knowledge and skills, but they are also learning how to work alongside others within complex and dynamic situations… From any vantage point, engagement in authentic work has a powerful influence on student learning. (p. 134)

Where engagement is lacking, learning is compromised. Students can become demotivated and disengaged (Dornan et al., 2007; Pratt et al., 2009; Roff et al., 2005). Orienting the students to a clinical setting and providing clear expectations is also an important step clinical instructors should take to reduce students' fears and facilitate a positive learning experience.

FACILITATING LEARNING

Effective clinical teachers guide students in the development of self-directed learning. "As there are stages in self-directed learning, so there are appropriate models of teaching for each stage" (Grow, 1991/1996). These stages (Dependent, Interested, Involved, and Self-Directed) and the corresponding levels of instructor involvement (Expert, Motivator, Facilitator, and Consultant) are illustrated in Figure 7.1. The Dependent student initially relies on and looks to the instructor for direction and expertise. As the learner transitions to the Interested student, the instructor fosters motivation in order for the student to become even more involved in his or her own learning (Motivated student). At this point, the instructor is facilitating learning to the point at which the student takes more

FIGURE 7.1

In the Staged Self-Directed Learning Model, the Instructor Ideally Matches the Stage of Learning to Prepare the Learner to Advance to Self-Directed Learning (Grow, 1991/1996)

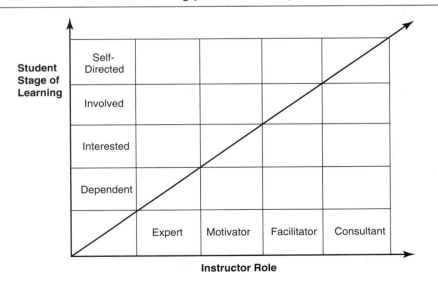

Instructor Role

responsibility and the instructor is acting as a consultant. The student is then prepared for lifelong learning; he or she is a Self-Directed student who can take the initiative, with or without the help of others, in diagnosing their learning needs, formulating learning goals, identifying human and material resources for learning, choosing and implementing appropriate learning strategies, and evaluating learning outcomes (Knowles, 1975, p. 18).

As discussed in chapter 3, it is imperative that today's health care workers become lifelong learners.

In an ideal situation, the instructor matches his or her style of teaching with the students' level of learning. For example, when students are dependent, the instructor coaches them in retrieving or activating knowledge. The instructor, in the role of the expert, may coach the students in the demonstration of particular skills. Immediate feedback is important at this stage, to overcome deficiencies, build self-confidence, and move the students to the Interested level. Allowing the students to gain insight into their own learning helps those who are in the Dependent stage begin to take responsibility for their own learning. Students can set their own learning goals even while at the Dependent level. Ways to interact with students at various levels are discussed later in this chapter.

In assessing students, the instructor needs to determine any gaps in knowledge and skill and any attitude problems (Kilminster & Jolly, 2000). As Lacasse et al. (2009) discussed, an educational diagnosis offers a way to manage a learner who may have attitude problems. They suggested first determining whether the problem lies in the learner's environment. Is the student facing personal, familial, or social problems? Does the problem lie in personal challenges, such as time management, organizational or study skills, or unfamiliarity with available resources? Does the student face frustration at the clinical site because of problems related to staffing and/or his or her role within the site? As we have stated, learning does not happen in isolation. It is the instructor's role to help the student toward resolution of these problems to facilitate learning. If the problem is frustration or lack of motivation for learning, then the instructor should reevaluate the student's level of learning. At the end of this chapter we present some well-established strategies for teaching in the clinical setting that offer ways to engage the learner.

EVALUATION

Clinical evaluation provides students with insight into their growth and performance. Although it is time consuming and often difficult, it is essential, because it provides direction, can enhance confidence and motivation, and serves as a tool for grading or assessment.

Evaluation in a clinical setting can be formal or informal, summative or formative, norm referenced or criterion referenced. Student knowledge, skills, and professionalism can be evaluated. Formative feedback is ongoing and can be given throughout the course of the day or clinical rotation. Evaluation in the clinical context can be written or spoken, and one of the benefits of formative evaluation as feedback to the students is that it is specific and timely. It allows for students to address weaknesses in a timely fashion (if necessary), and constructive criticism can increase confidence and motivation for learning (Clynes & Rattery, 2008; Dornan et al., 2007). A successful structure for clinical evaluation, the "One-Minute Preceptor," is presented in the next section.

It is helpful for the clinical instructor to keep written records of any feedback given, if possible, even if it is only in the form of daily notes on student performance. These notes on formative evaluation can transition into summative evaluations. Summative evaluations take place at the end of the clinical attachment and examine whether the objectives or outcomes for the attachment have been met.

Norm-referenced and criterion-referenced evaluations measure student performance against, respectively, a group or a set of performance criteria. Criterion-referenced evaluations are described in the "Competency-Based Methods of Learning" section. Many instructors will use a combination of these evaluation methods in the clinical setting.

SPECIFIC TECHNIQUES

The One-Minute Preceptor

The One-Minute Preceptor is a well-known and widely researched teaching strategy that can be used in the clinical setting (Irby & Wilkerson, 2008; Neher, Gordon, Meyer, & Stevens, 1992; Salerno, O'Malley, Pangaro, Wheeler, & Jackson, 2002). Clinical instructors use five microskills to assess the student using the One-Minute Preceptor (Neher, Gordon, Meyer, & Stevens, 1992):

1. Get a commitment.
2. Probe for supporting evidence (identify gaps in knowledge).
3. Teach general rules or principles.
4. Reinforce what was done right (give feedback).
5. Correct mistakes.

The One-Minute Preceptor model has the instructor ask questions in a nonthreatening way to engage the learner and provide immediate feedback. The student presents a clinical case to the instructor, and the instructor probes the student to expose his or her thinking by asking the following question back to the student: "What do *you* think is occurring in this case?" Such an approach by the instructor requires the student to process the information he or she just collected. The next step (probe for supporting evidence or alternative explanations) exposes the student's thinking patterns as he or she thinks aloud. Probing for supporting evidence is accomplished with questions such as "What led you to that diagnosis?" or "What would you do differently if the patient were pregnant?" These higher order questions challenge the learner in a nonthreatening manner while also motivating him or her.

At this point in the One-Minute Preceptor model the instructor teaches general rules or principles. Such rules are related to the case but also can be generalized to other situations. In describing the process of providing general rules to students, Neher et al. (1992) gave the example of saying to a student "It is well-established that ACE [angiotensin-converting enzyme] inhibitors reduce morbidity and prolong life in patients with dilated cardiomyopathy" as more appropriate than saying "This patient needs captopril." It is easy to see from this example how the student will gain more from the instructor's general rule than from a specific solution.

Next, the instructor offers constructive criticism and feedback to the student, including reinforcing what was done well. This time is also the opportunity to correct any mistakes and make specific recommendations for the student's improvement.

In short, the One-Minute Preceptor is a concise way to address student learning in the clinical setting.

SNAPPS

SNAPPS is a mnemonic device for **S**ummarize, **N**arrow possibilities, **A**nalyze, **P**robe, **P**lan, and **S**elect (Wolpaw, Wolpaw, & Papp, 2003). Used with medical students and based on real cases, this teaching tool is more learner driven than the One-Minute Preceptor, and it helps students organize their thinking and explore gaps in their understanding. This model can be used with students who are at a higher level of self-directed learning because it facilitates collaboration between the instructor and learner.

In the first step of SNAPPS the student presents a concise summary of the patient's history and physical examination. This summary should be no longer than 3 minutes and should provide only pertinent information. The second step of SNAPPS, narrow possibilities, is where the student presents two or three relevant possibilities of differential diagnoses. This is similar to the commitment stage of the One-Minute Preceptor. The student would next analyze these possibilities by comparing and contrasting the differentials. Such analysis demands a higher order of thinking from the learner and will allow the instructor a good view of the student's knowledge base. The fourth step allows the student to probe the instructor by asking questions. These questions may address uncertainties the student has in regard to the case, but the fact that the student generates the questions in this step makes the SNAPPS model more learner centered. Because the student is more involved with determining the learning issue, SNAPPS fosters the development of self-directed learning. The fifth step is to plan the clinical management of the patient, and the sixth and final step is fully self-directed learning in which the student must select a case-related learning issue.

This learner-centered model requires commitment on behalf of the learner and instructor. The Alberta Rural Physician Action Plan offers a resourceful Web site (http://www.practicalprof.ab.ca) with details about this and other effective teaching methods. The site includes short videos demonstrating both the One-Minute Preceptor and the SNAPPS model.

Competency-Based Methods of Learning

Educators of health care workers are challenged to find learning experiences that foster the integration of the essential knowledge, skills, and attitudes their students will need for the workplace. Education has traditionally been subject centered, aiming to convey a broad base of knowledge. Furthermore, evaluation through written testing may not adequately measure the learner's ability to perform the requisite skills. Even with a practical component, clinical rotations may not correspond with the classroom content and thus assessment may not adequately measure attitudes and skills. Traditionally, prepared students are expected to effectively do a job by drawing on the broad knowledge base covered in their education.

Competency-based learning is a student-centered teaching learning strategy that prepares health care workers in essential knowledge, skills (or practice), and attitudes to perform a particular job or function. This teaching learning strategy purports that, in order to thoroughly prepare a student for the job to be accomplished, health care worker educators must teach and evaluate skills and attitudes as well as knowledge.

Although it is important for students in all practice disciplines to display competence, it is imperative that health care workers be prepared to safely and effectively perform their work. A key to competency-based learning is that the role of the health care worker be clearly identified and relevant to the health of the community that will be served. This role, or professional profile, has a set of competencies that ensures that health care workers are prepared to address the problems commonly seen in the context of their work. *Competencies* have been defined as "what students will demonstrate by way of workplace attributes and profession-specific skills" (A. B. Voorhees, 2001, p. 87). These competencies are established through careful analysis of the specific tasks to be completed in the safe and effective performance of this work. Figure 7.2 illustrates how knowledge, skills, and attitudes form a foundation for the roles of health care workers.

A *task analysis table* is a way of organizing the broad tasks that comprise the competencies needed to acquire the requisite knowledge, attitudes and skills. Table 7.1 shows a sample task analysis table (from the Ethiopia Public Health Training Initiative Module on Diarrheal Disease; see chap. 10, this volume, for more on the Public Health Training Initiative). Note that information in the table is carefully arranged in sequential order. The identified task for this module is for the health care worker to "correctly identify and effectively manage diarrheal cases as well as prevent and control diarrheal disease." From an educational point of view, this task is too broad to be useful; further analysis is needed. It is therefore broken down in the task analysis table into the knowledge, skills (or practice), and attitude related to this area of competency. This clear description of the educational needs allows both the students and the teachers to understand their roles and expectations.

FIGURE 7.2

Knowledge, Attitudes and Skills as the Foundation of a Role

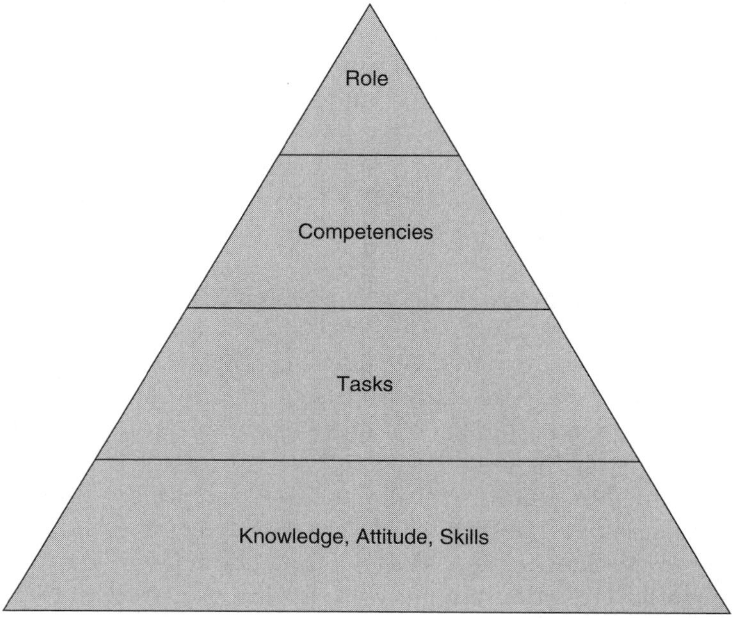

To further clarify expectations, in competency-based learning the out-comes are clearly stated through the use of measurable, student-centered learning objectives. These objectives "provide students with a clear map and the navigational tools needed to move expeditiously toward their goals" (R. A. Voorhees, 2001, p. 11; for a discussion on writing clear objectives, see chap. 8, this volume).

Cleary stated objectives allow students to measure their progress in mas-tering the material. *Mastery learning*, whereby students are given the opportu-nity to master the task at hand, is another key element of competency-based learning. Look again at Table 7.1. One of the competencies stated as an objective is for the Ethiopian health officer and medical laboratory technician to be able to carry out macro- and microscopic examination of a stool sample and identify the causative organism. By using the Checklist for Methylene Blue Fecal Smear Preparation (see Table 7.2), the student and instructor evaluate the student's performance objectively. This checklist is an example of a navigational tool that allows the learner to attain a certain competency level. The teacher acts as a facilitator by providing these tools, and the student is given ample opportunity to master the skills.

TABLE 7.1

TASK ANALYSIS TABLE FOR PRACTICE OBJECTIVES AND ESSENTIAL TASKS OF A HEALTH CENTER TEAM

1. Demonstrate the Process of Assessing a Child With Diarrhea and Identify Possible Complications

Health Officer Competencies	Essential Knowledge and Attitudes
1. Take an appropriate history and perform proper physical examination[a]	Concepts of good interviewing technique:
SKILLS	▪ 2-way communication
1.1 Conduct a history-taking interview using effective communication skills.	▪ Active listening
1.2 Follow a recommended sequence for taking a complete pediatric medical history.	▪ Open-ended questions
1.2.1 Patient identification information:	▪ Awareness of communication barriers
▪ Date of visit, name, address, sex, date of birth, age, birth order, other siblings	Causes and risk factors of diarrheal diseases
1.2.2 Review previous illnesses of each body system.	Magnitude and contribution of diarrheal disease to overall health problems, locally and nationally
1.2.3 Past medical history, including allergies, immunizations.	Preparation and use of the equipment for doing a pediatric physical examination
1.3 Perform proper physical examination:	Technique for handling infants and children to facilitate examination and promote child comfort
1.3.1 General appearance: State of health, state of nutrition, behavior, mental state	Manifestations and complications of diarrheal disease
1.3.2 Measurement: Height, weight, and arm circumference; Development: Social, language	
1.3.3 Skin: turgor, lesions, rash or sores	
1.3.4 HEENT: Fontanel; Eyes for tears, sunken; Mouth, mucous membranes	
1.3.5 Neck: Rigidity, ability to move neck	
1.3.6 Respiratory System	
1.3.7 Cardiac System	
1.3.8 Abdomen	
1.3.9 Extremities	

(Continued)

TABLE 7.1 (Continued)

TASK ANALYSIS TABLE FOR PRACTICE OBJECTIVES AND ESSENTIAL TASKS OF A HEALTH CENTER TEAM

2. Demonstrate How to Do Macro- and Microscopic Examination of the Stool in Case of Diarrheal Diseases

Health Officer and Med-Lab Tech Competencies	Essential Knowledge and Attitudes
1. Carry out macro- and microscopic examination of the stool sample and identify the organism	Types of diarrhea
SKILLS	Causes and risk factors of diarrheal diseases
1.1 Investigate macroscopically and microscopically.	Magnitude and contribution of diarrheal disease to overall health problems, locally and nationally
1.2 Record and report results of findings.	
1.3 Demonstrate precautions to be taken when handling specimens.	Occupational health regulations for handling specimens

aStudent performance can be evaluated through the use of a competency skills checklist.

Note. HEENT=head, eyes, ears, nose, and throat. From "Module on Diarrheal Disease for the Ethiopian Health Team," by T. Belachew, C. Jira, K. Faris, G. Makete, T. Asres, and H. Argaw, 2005, Ethiopia Public Health Training Initiative Module, Jimma University. Copyright 2005 by the Carter Center, Atlanta, GA. Reprinted with permission.

Table 7.2

CHECKLIST FOR METHYLENE BLUE FECAL SMEAR PREPARATION

Student demonstrates competency in each of the following:

Step	Procedure	Yes	No	N/A
1	Assembles all materials.[a]			
2	Places a drop of methylene blue at the center of the slide.			
3	Mixes a small amount of stool with the stain.			
4	Covers it with a glass.			
5	Examines the entire preparation using the 40X objective for fecal mononuclear (not lobed) and polymorphonuclear (a nucleus with two or more lobes) leukocytes.			
6	Adequately interprets slide.			
7	Reports and records results accurately.			
8	Cleans up station.			

[a] Materials needed: methylene blue staining solution, slide, cover glass, microscope, applicator stick and Pasteur pipette.

As one can see in Figure 7.3, which depicts the cycle for mastery learning, it is the teacher's role to ensure that the learning program provides the appropriate learning opportunities. The division of the job into competencies helps develop a list of learning objectives, and that in turn suggests the more appropriate type of learning strategy. The teaching learning strategies, therefore, are selected to help develop the student's competencies. Returning to the example from the Ethiopia Public Health Training Initiative, the teaching learning strategy for the development of laboratory competencies would be a practical session in which students could use the materials and the Checklist for the Methylene Blue Fecal Smear Preparation, whereas the task "Conduct a history-taking interview using effective communication skills" might best be fostered through a role play or observed interview (for more on role playing and observed interviews, see chap. 6, this volume).

Other examples of competency-based learning methods, in addition to checklists for learning, are Observed Structured Clinical Examinations (OSCE), patient simulations, and observation of real patient encounters. Competency-based learning methods are effectively used in the development of student portfolios, where students keep track of their progress. Competency-based portfolios are more than just logs in which students count numbers of procedures. Dannefer and Henson (2007) reported the successful use of a portfolio approach to competency-based assessment. They identified nine competencies for their students: (a) research, (b) medical knowledge, (c) communication, (d) professionalism, (e) clinical skills, (f) clinical reasoning, (g) health care systems, (h) personal development, and (i) reflective practice. Competencies are verified through the use of a variety of evaluative tools that are developed into a database that provides evidence of progression.

FIGURE 7.3

The Cycle for Mastery Learning

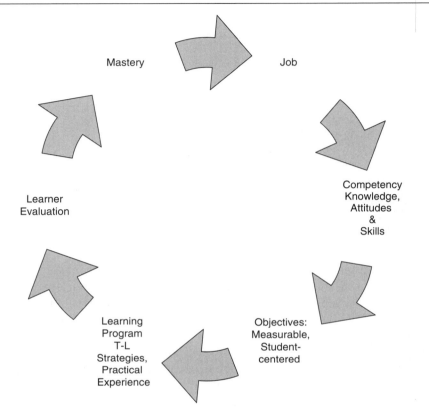

Sharing clearly stated and measurable objectives with students shifts the focus to student performance and away from instructional delivery (R.A. Voorhees, 2001). Much of the responsibility for progress in learning also shifts from faculty to student. As a result, competency-based learning can enhance students' motivation for learning and promote self-directed learning (Zimmerman & Dibenedetto, 2008). However, the competencies and objectives are narrowly defined and thus may not fully reflect the complex nature of the full role of the health care worker. It is important for the instructor to assist the learner in making connections and applications among and between competencies.

Competency-based learning has much to offer in the educational preparation of health care workers. It can be an effective, objective, and transparent teaching learning strategy, especially when used in conjunction with other strategies.

REFERENCES

Belachew, T., Jira, C., Faris, K., Mekete, G., Asres, T., & Argaw, H. (2005). *Module on diarrheal disease for the Ethiopian Health Team*. Unpublished document, Jimma University, Oromia Region, Jimma Zone, Ethiopia.

Bradshaw, M. (2011). Philosophical approaches to clinical instruction. In M. Bradshaw & A. Lowenstein (Eds.), *Innovative teaching strategies in nursing and related health professions* (5th ed., pp. 397–403). Sudbury, MA: Jones & Bartlett.

Clynes, M., & Rattery, S. (2008). Feedback: An essential element of student learning in clinical practice. *Nurse Education in Practice, 8*, 405–411. doi:10.1016/j.profnurs.2007.01.013

Dannefer, E., & Henson, L. (2007). The portfolio approach to competency-based assessment at the Cleveland Clinic Lerner College of Medicine. *Academic Medicine, 82*, 493–502.

Dornan, T., Boshuizen, H., King, N., & Scherpbier, A. (2007). Experience-based learning: A model linking the processes and outcomes of medical students' workplace learning. *Medical Education, 41*, 84–91. doi:10.1111/j.1365-2929.2006.02652.x

Grow, G. O. (1996). Teaching learners to be self-directed. *Adult Education Quarterly, 41*, 125–149. Retrieved from http://www.longleaf.net/ggrow (Original work published 1991)

Irby, I. M., & Wilkerson, L. (2008). Teaching when time is limited. *British Medical Journal, 336*. Retrieved from http://www.bmj.com/cgi/content/extract/336/7640/384

Kilminster, S., & Jolly, B. (2000). Effective supervision in clinical practice settings: A literature review. *Medical Education, 34*, , 827–840.

Knowles, M. (1975). *Self-directed learning. A guide for learners and teachers*. Englewood Cliffs, NJ: Cambridge Adult Education.

Lacasse, M., Lee, S., Ghavam-Rassoul, A., & Batty, H. (2009). Integrating teaching into the busy resident schedule: A learner-centered approach to raise efficiency (L-CARE) in clinical teaching. *Medical Teacher, 31*, e507–e513. Retrieved from http://www.informaworld.com/10.3109/01421590902842409

Masunaga, H., & Hitchcock, M. (2010). Residents' and faculty's beliefs about the ideal clinical teacher. *Family Medicine, 42*, 116–120.

Molodysky, E. (2006). Identifying and training effective clinical teachers: New directions in clinical teacher training. *Australian Family Physician, 35*, 53–55.

Neher, J., Gordon, K., Meyer, B., & Stevens, N. (1992). A five-step "microskills" model of clinical teaching. *Journal of the American Board of Family Practice, 5*, 419–424.

Pratt, D., Harris, P., & Collins, J. (2009). The power of one: Looking beyond the teacher in clinical instruction. *Medical Teacher, 32*, 133–137.

Roff, S., McAleer, S., & Skinner, A. (2005). Development and validation of an instrument to measure the postgraduate clinical learning and teaching educational environment for hospital-based junior doctors in the UK. *Medical Teacher, 27*, 326–331.

Salerno, S., O'Malley, P., Pangaro, L., Wheeler, G., & Jackson, J. (2002). Faculty development seminars based on the one-minute preceptor improve feedback in the ambulatory setting. *Journal of General Internal Medicine, 17*, 779–787.

Sherbino, J., Bandiera, G., & Frank, J. (2008). Assessing competence in emergency medicine trainees: An overview of effective methodologies. *Canadian Journal of Emergency Medicine, 10*, 365–371.

Sutkin, G., Wagner, E., Harris, I., & Schiffer, R. (2008). What makes a good clinical teacher in medicine? A review of the literature. *Academic Medicine, 83*, 452–466. doi:10.1097/ACM.0b013e31816bee61

Voorhees, A. B. (2001). Creating and implementing competency-based learning models. In R. A. Voorhees (Ed.), *Measuring what matters: Competency-based learning models in higher education* (pp. 83–95). San Francisco, CA: Jossey-Bass.

Voorhees, R. A. (2001). Competency-based learning models: A necessary future. *New Directions for Institutional Research, 110,* 5. Retrieved from http://www.laspau.harvard.edu/idia/mecesup/readings/CDIO/Competency-BasedLearningModels.pdf

Wall, D., Clapham, M., Riquelme, A., Vieira, J., Cartmill, R., Aspegren, K., & Roff, S. (2009). Is PHEEM a multi-dimensional instrument? An international perspective. *Medical Teacher, 3,* e521–e527. doi:10.3109/01421590903095528

Wolpaw, T. M., Wolpaw, D. R., & Papp, K. K. (2003). SNAPPS: A learner-centered model for outpatient education. *Academic Medicine, 78,* 893–898.

Zimmerman, B., & Dibenedetto, M. (2008). Mastery learning and assessment: Implications for students and teachers in an era of high-stakes testing. *Psychology in the Schools, 45,* 206–216.

8

Evaluation and Assessment

INTRODUCTION

All teachers encounter the need to assess the learning of students. Evaluation and assessment, which are essential skills in teacher preparation, take many forms, such as task performance, rating scales, essays, problem solving, and written test items, including multiple choice, sentence completion, and true–false items. The teacher must plan and prepare test items, rating scales, and other strategies to assess and evaluate students' learning in both classroom and clinical settings.

The focus of this chapter is on the principles of writing behavioral objectives, effective evaluation, and assessment of a student's performance and work. Learning how to assess students' skills and knowledge requires that the teacher be able to develop clear learning goals, behaviors, outcomes, and methods of evaluation. Oermann and Gaberson (2009) described the process of assessment as being essential to obtaining information about students and stated that it includes learning to judge performance, determine competence to practice, and making other decisions about students' knowledge and accomplishments. Assessment and evaluation provide a means of ensuring accountability for students' level of education and the quality of clinical services they will be able to provide.

DEFINITIONS

The words *evaluation* and *assessment* are often used interchangeably, although there are important distinctions in the use of the terms. Kizlik (2010) stated that assessment is a process "by which information is obtained relative to some known objective or goal," whereas evaluation is a process "that is designed to provide information that will help make a judgment about a given situation" (p. 1). Assessment involves the collection of data for the purpose of understanding an issue or a situation. Whether implicit or explicit, it is most helpful when it is related to a goal, objective, or outcome for which it was designed. *Measurement*, a related term, usually refers to the process of quantifying the data the teacher wants to assess, such as responses to test questions. Measurement can be accomplished without quantification but must have an instrument with qualitative properties, such as an accepted set of criteria or other measuring scale, which serves as a standard for the measurement process.

Evaluation is a more complex process in which the emphasis is on comparing data against a specific standard for the purpose of judging worth or quality (Huitt, Hummel, & Kaeck, 2001). Kizlik (2010) suggested that value is inherent to evaluation, because the process of evaluation provides information that will be essential in making a judgment about the situation. This judgment process, which is based on a standard set of criteria, is what makes evaluation so complex. "Teachers, in particular, are constantly evaluating students, and such evaluations are usually done in the context of comparisons between what was intended (learning, progress, behavior) and what was obtained" (Kizlik, 2010, p. 1).

PRINCIPLES OF GOOD EVALUATION

Oermann and Gaberson (2009, pp. 5–6) identified five principles of effective evaluation/assessment in a variety of settings. These principles are helpful when choosing assessment strategies and their implementation in classrooms, online courses, laboratories, and clinical settings:

1. Identify clearly the learning objectives and outcomes or competencies to be assessed or evaluated to determine the knowledge, skills, or performance to be assessed.
2. Match the assessment technique to the learning objective/outcome/goal.
3. Clearly explain to the student what is expected, and provide feedback about progress.
4. Use multiple assessment techniques.
5. Keep in mind the limitations of assessment when judging or evaluating the results; information from one performance is only a sample of the student's overall performance.

CHARACTERISTICS OF LEARNING

Learning is often described as being passive or active. *Passive learning* is described as teacher focused, whereas active learning involves both students and the teacher. According to studies ("Passive vs. active learning," 2001) that have focused on passive versus active learning, the retention rates for adults over a 3-day time period were reported as follows:

- 10% of what is read
- 20% of what is heard

- 30% of what is seen
- 50% of what is seen and heard
- 70% of what is said
- 90% of what is said and done

The take-home message for both teachers and learners is that adults can learn by combinations of listening, watching, and reading, but they learn best by being involved in the whole learning process in which both students and teachers actively participate.

Effective evaluation of the student's learning can yield feedback that will help both teacher and student improve their teaching and learning skills. Learning is complex, multidimensional, and integrated, and it is revealed over time. Effective evaluation should reflect the intent of what has been taught.

The Intent of Teaching: Students Learning

The intent of one's teaching is reflected in the goals and outcomes that are set for learners. Good evaluation assesses the students' learning and is used to improve the teacher's approaches to instruction. These approaches often reflect the types of learning the teacher prefers, values the most, and expects from students. One's values drive what and how one teaches and evaluates. Palmer (1998) stated that "We teach who we are," meaning that the teacher's values enter into every aspect of the teaching learning process, including assessment and evaluation. "Structuring learning experiences are at the heart of teaching and creating an educational process for every student" (Murray, 1989, p. 199).

Evaluation of students focuses on the levels of learning that are valued or expected in students and facilitates student growth and improvement. It includes not only what students know but also what they can do. Evaluation that is ongoing provides past and current performance data on students' progress and reflects the intent of the teaching. Clearly presenting the intent of the teaching provides structure and direction for students. It also helps the teacher choose appropriate instruction strategies. Sharing with students the intent and the teaching processes, including selected teaching strategies and expected learning experiences, prepares the students for the learning experiences to come, including assessment and evaluation.

Strategies for Identifying the Intent of Teaching

Several strategies are commonly used to identify the intent of teaching. One of the oldest and most common is *behavioral objectives*. Tyler (1949), in his seminal book *Basic Principles of Curriculum and Instruction*, focused on what was then called *product-oriented curriculum building*. He clearly described how to select learning experiences that are most likely to be useful in attaining behavioral learning objectives that can be measured against assessment criteria. Not all objectives are stated in behavioral terms. In general, the intent of what is being taught, and the accomplishments the teacher expects of the students, often can be expressed in specific, operational statements (Rossi & Freeman, 1985).

The intent of the teaching can also be stated as *goals* or *ends in view*, which are expressed through statements that are usually more general and abstract yet still focus on the desired student outcomes (Rossi & Freeman, 1985). This approach guides the learners in becoming actively engaged in thinking about the relationships between the specific topic being studied and the broader landscape of thought and action.

A third way for teachers to make the intent of their teaching known is through the use of *stated purposes*. Carefully stated purposes provide reasons why something exists or is done. Purposes may be stated as teachers' expectations of what students should or could be able to learn.

The final and more recent manner of expressing the intent of teaching and learning expectations is through the use of *outcomes*. Outcomes are stated in the form of the end result, the long-term effect that the teacher can assess with qualitative and/or quantitative methods. Some teachers qualify outcomes by referring to them as *desired outcomes*. Desired outcomes may be knowledge, selected skills, performance of specified tasks, or particular attitudes which are stated in the form of results or effects that can be assessed.

Levels of Theory and Learning

Regardless of whether the teacher chooses to state the intent of teaching in the form of objectives, goals, ends-in-view, purposes, or desired outcomes, the students need clear directions related to the level of learning that is expected of them; for example, is the intent for the students to name or categorize discrete items, or to relate several things or concepts, or to relate one situation with another, or to conceptualize and produce situations? Em Bevis (1978), in her now-classic book *Curriculum Building in Nursing: A Process*, described levels of learning in which she adapted Dickoff, James, and Wiedenbach's (1968) four levels of theory development for use in curriculum development and teaching learning processes. In an updated edition of her book, Bevis (1989) suggested that "The 4 levels provide help for writing course and learning activity objectives and are helpful in deriving evaluation criteria" (p. 23). These four levels are described in the following sections.

Level 1: Factor isolating. Level 1 is the most basic stage, the simplest type of activity, which involves naming, labeling, classifying, or categorizing. It concerns the process of separating discrete items by classifying them into similar or different categories. "Name the instruments used to measure blood pressure" would be an example of a Level 1 activity.

Level 2: Factor relating. Level 2 is the second stage of complexity and involves relating factors through the teaching learning process of depicting, describing, or relating. "This level describes or depicts how one single-named and classified thing (factor) relates to another single-named and classified thing (factor)" (Bevis, 1989, p. 23). Level 2 involves knowing how items relate to each other. An example might be asking a student to describe the differences between a Level 1 task and a Level 2 task.

Level 3: Situation related. At Level 3, the degree of complexity has increased to involve the relationship of situations. This process includes relating one situation to another, such as in demonstrating the stain used for identifying the tubercle bacilli and explaining why another stain would not be applicable in that situation (i.e., if one suspected a diagnosis of tuberculosis). Level 3 also involves the process of comparing causal-connecting statements or situations, such as realizing that if the water main is broken at the place where it enters the community health center, then there can be no hand-washing, laundry, or any other activity that requires water within the building.

Level 4: Situation producing. Level 4 is the highest level of complexity and specifies how situations may be produced or made to occur. This high-level teaching learning process involves conceptualization of a situation or project and articulation of how to make it happen. A situation-producing activity includes the following five elements: (a) who does the activity; (b) who receives the activity; (c) what comprises the environment; (d) what guides the production of the situation; and (e) what energy sources, such as finances, materials, and human power, are available. An example Level 4 project might be to modify a community health center to make the facility culturally congruent for its service sector as well as family and patient oriented.

Although the levels-of-theory-and-learning model was developed and described by nurse theorists and educators, as applied to assessment and evaluation it is applicable to all health-related disciplines. In Table 8.1 we provide sample stem words that can be used as verbs to articulate an appropriate level of learning action.

TABLE 8.1

LEVELS OF THEORY AND LEARNING

Level 1: Factor isolating	Level 2: Factor relating	Level 3: Situation relating	Level 4: Situation producing
Perceive	Describe	Interpret	Use
Label	Relate factors	Explain	Plan
Classify	Draw/sketch	Order	Design
Identify	Discuss	Theorize	Organize
Record	Translate	Predict	Create
Recall	Diagram	Compare	Compose
Restate	Analyze factors	Rate	Choose
Report	Categorize	Apprise	Index
Examine	Define	Relate situations	Test
		Synthesize	Solve
		Critique	Practice
		Combine	Substitute
		Systematize	Build
			Vary
			Implement

Adapted from Bevis (1978).

WRITING GOALS, OUTCOMES, AND OBJECTIVES

Clearly defined goals, outcomes, and objectives serve several purposes. Davis (2001) identified the following three key aspects of goals and objectives:

1. They clarify intent of instruction for the teacher.
2. They communicate what students will accomplish.
3. They determine the appropriate content, learning activities, and assessment methods.

Goals are broadly stated and form the "big picture." Well-thought-out goals can have both content and noncontent components (Davis, 2001). For example, Harvard Medical School (2010) stated the following goal for its program in palliative care: "become expert in the clinical practice and teaching of comprehensive, interdisciplinary palliative care." The content goals listed on the site are clearly related to palliative care and include content on pain management, chronic illness, and grief, but to "become expert" in interdisciplinary care would undoubtedly require a goal related to excellence in communication and teamwork. This noncontent goal dictates course activities requiring students to work in groups.

The words *outcome* and *objective* are often used interchangeably. Both are used to convey educational aims; however, outcomes are generally broader and more student centered. They are stated in terms of achievement or results. Whereas objectives can be seen in terms of the educational *process*, outcomes place an emphasis on the *product* (Harden, 2002). Outcomes are seen as student centered, whereas objectives reflect the "teaching intentions" or the "subject content the teacher intends to cover" (University of Connecticut, n.d., p. 1) and can therefore be seen as subject or teacher centered. Objectives are written as intended consequences that imply learning, whereas outcomes are stated as results of the course of study.

Objectives are succinct, clear statements that describe the intention of instruction in terms of knowledge, skills, and attitudes the students will exhibit. Although objectives reflect broader goals, well-written objectives provide evidence of learning. Bloom (1984) identified three types of learning objectives: (a) cognitive (knowing), (b) behavioral (doing), and (c) affective (feeling or caring).

Objectives are most commonly written for the cognitive and behavioral domains because they are easier to measure than those for the affective domain. Cognitive objectives can be measured with examinations, and behavioral objectives can be measured through demonstrations. As discussed elsewhere in this book (chap. 7), professional competencies in terms of communication, appearance, and teamwork are part of the affective domain (Davis, 1981; Masin, 2002). The affective domain, even the "subtle and complex construct" of professionalism, "does not reduce easily to numerical scales" (Ginsburg, Regehr, & Mylopoulos, 2009, p. 414). Just because the affective domain is more difficult to assess than the cognitive and behavioral domains does not mean it should be overlooked. In fact, there is a danger that students may not realize the value of their feelings and attitudes if this domain is not explicitly identified by the instructor. (See also chap. 5, this volume, for a discussion of teaching knowledge, skills, and attitudes, and chap. 7. this volume, for a discussion of competency-based learning.)

Mager (1997) identified three components of a well-written objective:

1. The *condition* under which the performance must occur. Example: "By the end of the semester, the student will be able discuss cultural issues related to death and dying."
2. The *performance verb*, that is, what it is the student must do. Example: "Given a stethoscope and blood pressure cuff, the student will be able manually interpret a patient's blood pressure accurately."
3. The *criteria* by which the performance is assessed. Example: "When participating in interdisciplinary team meetings, the student will describe the roles of the other team members."

The condition is often consistent ("By the end of the semester . . .") and is not always stated with each objective.

Levels of Learning

The verb indicates the level of the objective. Bloom's (1984) taxonomy is widely used for articulating cognitive levels. Bloom identified six categories: (a) knowledge, (b) comprehension, (c) application, (d) analysis, (e) synthesis, and (f) evaluation. Knowledge is considered a "lower level." The learner is expected to "list" or "recall" certain facts. A higher cognitive level, such as analysis, would require the learner to differentiate or compare and contrast concepts.

Examples of verbs commonly used in each of the cognitive categories are presented in Table 8.2.

TABLE 8.2

COMMONLY USED VERBS

Category (noun)	Description (verb)	Key words
Knowledge	Recall or remember	Defines, describes, identifies, labels, lists, matches, names
Comprehension	Understanding the meaning	Classifies, discusses, distinguishes, estimates, explains, gives examples, paraphrases, summarizes
Application	Using or applying information	Applies, computes, predicts, demonstrates, modifies, uses
Analysis	Distinguish components	Analyzes, compares, contrasts, diagrams, differentiates, discriminates,
Synthesis	Evaluating; rearranging components to make a whole	Composes, creates, designs, explains, generates, plans, writes.
Evaluation	Creating a new product or idea	Appraises, concludes, critiques, defends, evaluates, judges

Note. From *Bloom's Taxonomy Verbs*, *http://www.teach-nology.com/worksheets/time_savers/bloom*, 2010. Copyright 2010 by Teachnology, Inc. Adapted with permission.

RELATING ASSESSMENT TO LEARNING

It is important to assess student learning in the classroom as well as in the clinical or laboratory setting. Assessment in the clinical setting was discussed in chapter 7. The plan for assessment is commonly included in the course syllabus or outline given to the students and may include a weighted breakdown of each assignment or a blueprint. A plan for grading and a blueprint, which communicate to students how performance will be assessed, are illustrated in Exhibit 8.1 and Table 8.3, respectively. By listing each objective in the left column, and the method of assessment (assignments, written examinations and practical examinations) across the top, a blueprint can ensure that all objectives are being assessed through a variety of appropriate methods. A blueprint also can determine whether the means of assessment are aligned with the objective. Whereas knowledge can be assessed with a written examination, skills may best be assessed with a practical examination, such as an Observed Structured Clinical Examination (OSCE). OSCE is a structured evaluation of clinical performance through the use of planned stations or simulated patient scenarios.

EXHIBIT 8.1

Plan for Grading

1. Episodic SOAP notes and case presentation	15%
2. Quizzes (5 worth 5 per cent each)	25%
3. Midterm examination	15%
4. Final exam	15%
5. Observed structured clinical examination	30%

Note. SOAP = subjective, objective, assessment, plan.

TABLE 8.3

A PARTIAL LIST OF OBJECTIVES AND ASSESSMENT METHODS FOR A HEALTH ASSESSMENT COURSE

Course Objective	Written Examination	Observed Structured Clinical Examination	Submitted Charting/SOAP Notes
1. Accurately and succinctly record history and physical findings and management plan	✓	✓	✓
2. Present assessment findings and management plan in an informed and professional manner		✓	✓
3. Utilize principles and techniques of physical examination for health assessment of clients	✓	✓	

Note. SOAP = subjective, objective, assessment, plan.
Adapted From *Nursing Education: Foundations for Practice Excellence*, by B. Moyer and R. Wittmann-Price, 2008, Philadelphia, PA: F.A. Davis.

Writing and Evaluating Test Questions

Objective test questions have been a major part of educational experiences for many years. Recognizing the usefulness of testing and evaluating with objective test questions, understanding the limitations of such testing, and being able to construct objective test questions are useful skills for teachers. Evaluating learning outcomes requires that one be able to use a variety of evaluation strategies and questions to obtain indicators of how well students are meeting the stated goals and objectives.

Planning

When planning a test, there are many questions to consider. How many questions are required for each topic or unit? How long will the test be? How long will the students have to take the test? It is sometimes helpful to use a blueprint similar to that in Table 8.3. List the units or topics to be covered in the test in the left column, and list the level of knowing across the top (Moyer & Wittmann-Price, 2008). In doing this, consider the *type* of learning you seek from the students. Should the students memorize drug names? Should they be able to select the correct medication when presented with a case study? Should they analyze or evaluate a situation? The different levels of knowing will direct the type of questions you will develop.

Review the learning objectives to determine what material will be covered in the test. In planning for the test, the instructor must also determine the type (or types) of questions as well as how many questions to include. Consider the reading level of the students taking the examination. In general, it should take 1 minute for a student to answer one multiple-choice or two true–false questions (DeYoung, 2003). This rule would not apply to questions with longer reading sections or that require complex calculations.

Types of Questions

Multiple-choice, true–false, and matching questions are the most frequently used type of test items. The benefit of these is that they can be easier to score than short answer or essay questions; however, it can be difficult to compose short questions that evaluate higher order learning. In any case, avoid the words *always* and *never*, and limit the use of *sometimes* and *often*.

Multiple-choice questions have two parts: (a) stems and (b) options. The options include a correct answer and distracters (incorrect answers).

The following are some helpful hints when writing stems:

1. The stem should be concise.
2. Word stems should be in the positive form (e.g., "Which of the following is an example of …?") rather than the negative form (e.g., "Which of the following is **not** …?").
3. The stem should be grammatically correct and consistent with the distracters but should avoid irrelevant clues; for example:

The vector for schistosomiasis is a/an

  a. animal
  b. insect
  c. snail

The number and types of options may vary but should be grammatically consistent with the stem. The distracters "All of the above" and "None of the above" should rarely be used. Avoid using nonsensical, humorous, or impossible distracters. All should be realistic and of similar length. In cases of numerical answers, they should be mutually exclusive ("less than 10," "between 11 and 20") and in ascending or descending order. One-word answers can be placed in alphabetical order, as in the example just offered. That said, be sure the positions of the correct answers are varied. Students can recognize patterns or preferred answers (e.g., if b and c are the more common correct answers). See Exhibit 8.2 for examples of leveled questions.

True–false questions are designed to evaluate the student's ability to recognize facts or, at most, the relationships between concepts. They cannot evaluate higher order levels of learning. It is important that the question be clearly stated and unambiguous. A variation on the true–false question asks the student to explain why the correct response is "true" or "false." This technique can evaluate higher levels of learning but loses some of the objectivity and time-saving benefits.

Matching questions also test lower levels of learning. Matching questions normally appear as two lists or columns, with the stems on the left and the answer on the right. Be sure to include clear instructions that include whether an answer can be used more than once, or not at all. As with all questions, be sure there are no irrelevant clues, such as discrepancies between verb tenses or plural/singular clues. For examples of test questions see Zimmaro (2003). Here are some other things to consider when writing matching questions:

- They should have no fewer than 5 but no more than 10 items.
- Be sure the question with all stems and possible answers are on one page.
- Use single words or short phrases as answers.
- The lists should be homogeneous.

Short answer or essay questions test higher levels of knowing. They take less time to prepare but more time to answer and grade. Restricted-response answers place limitations on the response (Oermann & Gaberson, 2009). These types of questions can be used with case studies (see chap. 6, this volume). Before grading, one should write out a key for the correct response. Points can be assigned for partial and complete answers.

EVALUATING OUTCOMES

In addition to assessing the success of individual students, there are methods for overall evaluation of educational programs. One commonly used method is that of pass rates for standardized national qualification examinations.

EXHIBIT 8.2

Examples of Levels of Knowledge in Multiple-Choice Questions

Level 1, Knowledge (recall):
Malaria is a disease caused by

1. Virus
2. Ricketessia
3. Bacteria
4. Protozoa

Level 2, Comprehension:
Thick blood smear is more advantageous than thin blood smear in

1. Easy identification of parasites in blood film
2. Easy identification of plasmodia species in blood film
3. Taking less time for specimen processing

Level 3, Application:
An intravenous 600 mg quinine in 600 ml 5% dextrose in saline is ordered to run for 4 hours. Calculate the rate of flow (given 1 ml = 15 drops / min).

1. 38 drops/min
2. 162.5 drops/ min
3. 900 ml/min
4. 38 ml/min
5. 190 drop/min

Level 4, Analysis:
A patient arrives at the health center. He lives in a malarious area and reports a history of headaches, fever, and chills. He took two aspirin and is "feeling better now." The blood smear shows crescent-shaped gametocytes. What would this indicate?

1. The patient does not have malaria.
2. The patient has falciparum malaria.
3. The patient's malaria has resolved.
4. The slide should be repeated.

Standardized qualification examinations are required for licensure in many countries (the Australian Medical Council Examination, the National Council Licensure Examinations for Registered Nurses, the U.S. Medical Licensing Examination, and the South African Nursing Council Examination, to name a few). Another commonly used assessment strategy is to have an external examiner, a person from another institution or organization, evaluate individual students or entire programs. External examiners can monitor the assessment process (written examinations, clinical performance) of students. Reviewers can also certify a program or school by evaluating the faculty and full curriculum. This can lead to accreditation by educational or professional bodies. Where accreditation is required, students must graduate from accredited schools in order to qualify for licensure.

| LEARNING ACTIVITY 8.1 |
| DEVELOPING TEST QUESTIONS |

OVERVIEW

Objective test questions have been a major part of our educational experiences for many years. The results of these tests have made an impact on our lives, sometimes negative and sometimes positive. Recognizing the usefulness of testing and evaluating with objective test questions, understanding the limitations of such testing, and being able to construct objective test questions are useful skills for teachers. Evaluating learning outcomes requires that one be able to use a variety of evaluation strategies and questions to obtain indicators of how well students are meeting the stated goals and objectives. In this learning activity we discuss evaluation and how to write different types of questions, and we will practice writing and critiquing test questions. Add to the bottom of learning activity the following text:

DIRECTIONS

Following a brief presentation:

1. You will be asked to break into work groups of 5. Each group will be assigned a specific type of question.
   - Question types
     a. Multiple-choice test items
     b. True–false test items
     c. Matching test items
     d. Completion items
     e. Essay test items
     f. Problem-solving test items
2. Each group will do the following:
   a. Design a brief presentation on your assigned type of question using the information in the handout that you have read. Use flipchart paper and markers to prepare your presentation.
   b. Develop two sample questions.
   c. Present it to the larger group to be critiqued and discussed.

RESOURCES

Helpful resources for the preparation of examinations and test questions include the following:

Zimmaro, D. M. (2003). *Writing effective examinations*. Austin, TX: Measurement and Evaluation Center, The University of Texas. Retrieved from http://www.utexas.edu/academic/mec/research/pdf/writingexamshandout.pdf

Improving your test questions
http://www.oir.uiuc.edu/dme/exams/ITQ.html

Teaching tips: Test Item Writing
http://www.uab.edu/uasomume/cdm/test.htm

REFERENCES

Bevis, E. O. (1978). *Curriculum building in nursing: A process*. St. Louis, MO: Mosby.

Bevis, E. O. (1989). *Curriculum building in nursing: A process* (3rd ed.). Sudbury, MA: Jones & Bartlett.

Bloom, B. (1984). *Taxonomy of educational objectives*. New York, NY: Longman.

Davis, B. (2001). *Tools for teaching*. San Francisco: Jossey Bass.

Davis, C. (1981). Affective education for the health professions: Facilitating appropriate behavior. *Physical Therapy, 61,* 1587–1593.

DeYoung, S. (2003). *Teaching strategies for nurse educators*. Upper Saddle River, NJ: Pearson Education.

Dickoff, J., James, P., & Wiedenbach, E. (1968). Theory in practice discipline: Part 1. Practice oriented theory. *Nursing Research, 17,* 415–434.

Ginsburg, S., Regehr, G., & Mylopoulos, M. (2009). From behaviors to attributions: Further concerns regarding the evaluation of professionalism. *Medical Education, 43,* 414–425.

Harden, R. M. (2002). Learning outcomes and instructional objectives: Is there a difference? *Medical Teacher, 24,* 151–155. doi:10.1080/0142159022020687

Harvard Medical School. (n.d.). *Program in palliative care education and practice*. Retrieved from http://www.hms.harvard.edu/pallcare/pcep.htm#ProgramGoals

Huitt, W., Hummel, J., & Kaeck, D. (2001). *Assessment, measurement, evaluation, and research*. Retrieved from http://www.edpsycinteractive.org/topics/intro/sciknow.html

Kizlik, B. (2010). *Measurement, assessment, and evaluation in education*. Retrieved from http://www.adprima.com/measurement.htm

Mager, R. (1997). *Preparing instructional objectives: A critical tool in the development of effective instruction*. Atlanta, GA: Center for Effective Performance.

Masin, H. I. (2002). Education in the affective domain: A method/model for teaching professional behaviors in the classroom and during advisory sessions. *Journal of Physical Therapy Education, 16,* 37–45.

Moyer, B., & Wittmann-Price, R. (2008). *Nursing education: Foundations for practice excellence*. Philadelphia, PA: F.A. Davis.

Murray, J. P. (1989). Making the connection: Teacher–student interactions and learning experiences. In E. O. Bevis & J. Watson (Eds.), *Toward a caring curriculum: A new pedagogy for nursing* (pp. 189–215). New York, NY: National League for Nursing.

Oermann, M. H., & Gaberson, K. B. (2009). *Evaluation and testing in nursing education* (3rd ed.). New York, NY: Springer Publishing.

Palmer, P. J. (1998). *The courage to teach*. San Francisco, CA: Jossey-Bass.

Passive vs. active learning. (2001). Retrieved from http://www.justice.gov/adr/workplace/pdf/wp-reten.pdf

Rossi, P. H., & Freeman, H. E. (1985). *Evaluation: A systematic approach*. Beverly Hills, CA: Sage.

Tyler, R. W. (1949). *Basic principles of curriculum and instruction*. Chicago, IL: University of Chicago Press.

University of Connecticut. (n.d.). *How to write program objectives/outcomes*. Retrieved from http://assessment.uconn.edu/docs/HowToWriteObjectivesOutcomes.pdf

Zimmaro, D. M. (2003). *Writing effective examinations*. Austin, TX: Measurement and Evaluation Center, The University of Texas. Retrieved from http://www.utexas.edu/academic/mec/research/pdf/writingexamshandout.pdf

9

The Teacher as Leader, Role Model, and Mentor

Leadership theories have been evolving over the past 70 years and include trait, behaviorist, situational, and contingency theories; today, they have evolved into transactional and transformational theories (Bolden, Gosling, Marturano, & Dennison, 2003). As opposed to earlier years, when the "great man" theory (which described history as occurring through the actions of "great men") was dominant, today many women are in leadership positions, and multiple leadership theories exist.

Leadership theories continue to evolve and offer insights into the qualities of successful leaders who also become role models and mentors. Teachers are leaders, role models, and mentors to students who will become the leaders of the future. In this chapter we provide information on leadership theories and present selected leadership models and activities to evaluate and support growth as teachers who are leaders, role models, and mentors. Learning Activity 9.1, at the end of this chapter, will help you develop your vision statement as a teacher based on your best personal case as a leader.

LEADERSHIP THEORIES AND COMPETENCIES

Multiple theories, models, and competency frameworks define the leadership, management qualities, and competencies being used today. Bolden et al. (2003) conducted a review of leadership theories and competency frameworks to assist in the development of new frameworks for leadership. Their review reported on the evolution of leadership theory and competency frameworks over 70 years, ranging from the "great man" theory to the transactional and transformational theories of today.

Bolden et al. (2003) also conducted a search of leadership theories and identified seven models or schools of thought: (a) "great man" theories, (b) trait theories, (c) behaviorist theories, (d) situational leadership, (e) contingency theory,

(f) transactional theories, and (g) transformational theories. It is not the aim of this chapter to present all of these theories; instead, the purpose is to focus on transformational leadership needed for the complex world of today, including education and health in low-resource countries. The focus of transformational leadership in education is to bring about change and to envision and implement transformation through the roles of educator and mentor.

Bass (1985) investigated transactional and transformational leadership. He identified *superior leadership* as transformational leadership that occurs when leaders broaden and elevate the interests of their employees or students, when they generate awareness and acceptance of the purposes and mission of the group, and when they inspire their employees or students to look beyond their own self-interest for the good of the group. Transformational leaders achieve results through being charismatic and inspiring, meeting the emotional needs of employees, or by being intellectually stimulating. Teachers function as transformational leaders in education in their roles as teachers and mentors.

Kouzes and Posner (1995), in their book *The Leadership Challenge*, addressed the challenges leaders and teachers face to get extraordinary things done in many challenging situations and organizations. They described the current world situation as "encompassing new realities, whereby power has shifted: everyone is connected through technology, knowledge is essential, the world is fragmented, and there is a new search for meaning" (pp. xvii–xx).

Kouzes and Posner (1995, pp. 8–14) posited five fundamental practices of exemplary leadership that have created extraordinary results in a variety of settings, including education: (a) challenge the process, (b) inspire a shared vision, (c) enable others to act, (d) model the way, and (e) encourage the heart. The other common element in the success of these practices is a willingness to take risks. Challenging people and situations takes courage and leads to changes in the status quo. Challenges also lead to change, innovation, experiments, learning, and personal growth.

In the sections that follow, we explore these five fundamental practices of leadership and discuss how they fit into the education and preparation of health care workers.

CHALLENGING THE PROCESS

Challenging the process in teaching and learning requires one to be willing to explore new and different approaches to teaching and learning. Many challenges exist today in educational settings in regard to technology and other methods of teaching. To be considered competent, faculty and teachers are expected to stay current with changes, technology, teaching strategies, and research. Motivation, experimentation, taking risks, and learning from mistakes are needed if one wants to challenge current processes of teaching and learning.

As leaders, teachers search for opportunities to improve the status quo and to improve students' educational experiences. Leaders search for challenging opportunities to change, grow, innovate, and improve situations and organizations. Experimenting, taking risks, and learning from mistakes are part of the challenge. Health education faces the challenges of helping teachers of health care workers develop a variety of teaching methods, relate to students in different ways, and improve current educational and health care settings. Teachers must be willing to take risks and to innovate in the classrooms and clinical settings to educate health care workers.

Multiple innovative teaching approaches have been developed in the recent past and have been incorporated into health care worker education. Educational research is supporting the challenge of using active teaching learning strategies, online courses, small group work, and simulation and is challenging teachers to become competent in different active teaching learning strategies. Innovative teaching learning strategies are replacing the typical model of the traditional lecture, in which the teacher does most of the talking.

Essential activities that must be embraced to fulfill the commitment of challenging current educational processes include arousing an intrinsic motivation in oneself and others, balancing daily routines and change, exploring innovation and outside stimulation, learning from mistakes and encouraging others to do the same, promoting and trying new approaches, and making something happen.

The search for opportunities to improve the status quo—to grow, innovate, and improve—challenges the process. Leaders experiment, take risks, and learn from mistakes. Teachers face the challenge of developing a variety of instruction methods so they can relate to students in different ways and thus improve the educational institution. Teachers/mentors expect students/mentees to accomplish many things and to bring about change and improvement. Activities essential to fulfilling the commitment of challenging the process include the following:

- Motivating oneself and others
- Balancing the paradox of routine approaches and being willing to utilize new teaching methods and technology
- Looking for new, different, and stimulating teaching methods
- Learning from different situations and encouraging students and colleagues to do the same
- Promoting hardiness and fostering risk-taking to improve teaching and learning
- Making something happen (Kouzes & Posner, 1995, pp. 37–52)

INSPIRING A SHARED VISION

Teachers passionately believe they can make a difference. They envision the future, creating an ideal and unique image of what they do and what they can do to help others to become competent and successful. Teachers enlist others in the common vision by appealing to their values, interest, hopes, and dreams. One example of shared vision is currently found in nursing education. A new vision for nursing education and practice has recently been published: *Educating Nurses: A Call for Radical Transformation* (Benner, Sutphen, Leonard, & Day, 2009). The focus of the book is on challenging current practices and transforming nursing practice and education. Although the book focuses on nursing, its call for transformation is applicable to other health care worker programs that are working to transform education and practices to meet the needs for the future. Sharing this vision with and enlisting professionals in the fields of practice and education will lead to the needed changes so that these health care needs will be met. Professionals in the fields of education and practice recognize the need to update, change, and improve education and practice to adequately prepare health workers for a changing health care environment. This is essential in countries with both low and high levels of resources.

Change of this magnitude requires the involvement and commitment of health care workers, clinical agencies, physicians, and health care worker educational programs. Sharing a vision and designing health care for the future is the challenge at hand, and it requires change on many levels.

Leaders passionately believe that they can make a difference. They envision the future, creating an ideal and unique image of what they can help others and the organization to become. Leaders enlist others in the common vision by appealing to their values, interests, hopes, and dreams. Health science teachers act as role models, encourage students to create a vision of their career, and appeal to students to discover the common purpose of improving the health status of their clients. Several activities can help leaders inspire a shared vision:

- Imaging the ideal and intuiting the future
- Discovering and appealing to common goals and outcomes
- Communicating expressively, thereby bringing a shared vision to life in such a way that students can see themselves in it
- Sincerely believing in what you are saying and demonstrating your personal beliefs and vision (Kouzes & Posner, 1995, pp. 18, 91–120)

ENABLING OTHERS TO ACT

Leaders foster collaboration, build spirited teams, and actively involve others. They understand that mutual respect is what sustains extraordinary efforts, and they strive to create an atmosphere of trust and dignity. They strengthen others, making them feel capable and powerful. Teachers view learners/mentees as able, and they pursue "power with," not "power over," relationships. Active participatory approaches to teaching, learning, and mentoring help students and increase learning. The following strategies are essential to fulfilling a commitment to enabling others to act:

- Developing cooperative learning goals
- Seeking integrative solutions to problems

- Building trusting relationships
- Ensuring self-leadership by putting people in control of their own lives
- Providing choice
- Developing competence
- Offering visible support (Kouzes & Posner, 1995, pp. 18, 151–206)

MODELING THE WAY

Leaders establish principles concerning the way individuals should be treated and the way goals should be pursued. They create standards of excellence and then set an example for others to follow. Because the prospect of complex change can overwhelm people and stifle action, they set interim goals so that people can achieve small wins as they work toward larger goals. They work through the bureaucracy when it gets in the way of action. Leaders provide signposts or directions when people are unsure of where to go or how to get there. They create opportunities for victory and success. The following activities will help leaders who are committed to modeling the way:

- Clarifying personal values, beliefs, and goals of oneself and others
- Becoming unified in regard to shared values and paying attention to how you, students, and other health professionals and colleagues are living the values
- Achieving small wins that promote consistent progress and build commitment
- Sustaining commitment to the process as it works and improves
- Setting the example by behaving in ways that are consistent with shared values (Kouzes & Posner, 1995, pp. 18, 209, 241)

ENCOURAGING THE HEART

Accomplishing extraordinary things in educational organizations is hard work. To keep hope and determination alive, leaders recognize contributions that individuals make. In every winning team, the members need to share in the rewards of their efforts, so leaders celebrate accomplishments. They make people feel like heroes. Some ways of doing this include:

- Recognizing individual accomplishments
- Building self-confidence through high, yet realistic expectations
- Recognizing growth and performance of individuals and teams
- Being positive and hopeful
- Being personally involved
- Creating social support by building a community of teaching scholars (Kouzes & Posner, 1995, pp. 18, 269–290)

LEARNING ACTIVITY 9.1

**DEVELOPING PERSONAL AND PROFESSIONAL
LEADERSHIP ACTIVITIES**

Extraordinary changes do not happen without the active involvement and support of individuals who will be affected by the change. Creating cooperation and working as a team leads to change, not just the "personal best" of one person. Collaboration, as opposed to competition, leads to success in accomplishing goals. Leaders who collaborate and are supported by others perform better, promote trust, and work together to accomplish the desired outcomes.

ACTIVITY 1: READ THE FOLLOWING LETTER

Dear Honored Faculty Member:

Congratulations! You have been chosen "Leader of the Year." There will be a televised award dinner in your honor on Tuesday. In order to make this event really special, we need your help. How would you like to be recognized? Please share with us the words you would most like to hear used to describe you.

Thank you for all of your hard work!

ACTIVITY 2: RESPOND TO THE FOLLOWING ITEMS

1. Break into small groups of 4–6. Discuss Kouzes and Posner's 5 practices: (1) challenging the process; (2) inspiring a shared vision; (3) enabling others to act; (4) modeling the way; (5) encouraging the heart.
2. Discuss and describe how you would like to be recognized as a leader/teacher. Share characteristics of your favorite teacher or leader.
3. Discuss the characteristics needed in educational and health leaders to meet the health care needs of the population in your current environment.
4. Identify persons in your life that you view as successful leaders.
5. Share stories related to positive experiences with teachers/leaders.

ACTIVITY 3: WRITE BRIEF STATEMENTS

1. Based upon Kouzes and Posner's 5 leadership practices, describe how you will incorporate these practices into your role as teacher.
2. Write a short vision statement that will reflect who you want to be as a teacher.

REFERENCES

Bass, B. M. (1985). *Leadership and performance beyond expectations*. New York, NY: Free Press.

Benner, P., Sutphen, M., Leonard, V., & Day, L. (2009). *Educating nurses: A call for radical transformation*. San Francisco, CA: Jossey-Bass.

Bolden, R., Gosling, J., Marturano, A. & Dennison, P. (2003). *A review of leadership theory and competency frameworks*. Centre for Leadership Studies, University of Exeter, Exeter, England. Retrieved from http://centres.exeter.ac.uk/cls/research/abstract.php?id=29

Kouzes, J. M., & Posner, B. Z. (1995). *The leadership challenge*. San Francisco, CA: Jossey-Bass.

10

Training Health Care Professionals in Low-Resource Environments: Applying Active Teaching Learning Strategies in Ethiopia

THE ETHIOPIA PUBLIC HEALTH TRAINING INITIATIVE

As we have detailed throughout this book, the foundation of quality health care begins with properly trained health care professionals who are competent, versatile, and accessible. Training such health care workers is a large task, but an achievable one with the right approach, as evidenced in the preceding chapters. In the case of Ethiopia, training in health care has been a long road. As in other low-resource environments, life for the average Ethiopian family is challenging with the realities of health issues and health care grim. Compounding the limited availability of health care workers in rural areas is the stark void left by the migration of native skilled health care workers to other countries, with rural areas being hardest hit by the emigration of health professionals (Serneels et al., 2010).

A lack of health professionals is not specific to Ethiopia, though. The World Health Organization recently documented the critical shortage of global health care workers, particularly nurses (Chen et al., 2006). However, the shortage of health professionals is most severe in the poorest countries, especially sub-Saharan Africa. Without these workers, people suffer daily, without aid for fully preventable maladies such as diarrhea, malnutrition, malaria, and HIV/AIDS (Carlson, 2007). This very urgent need to boost the numbers of health workers globally is an area The Carter Center addresses with its Ethiopia Public Health Training Initiative (EPHTI).

Less than half of Ethiopia's population has access to modern health services, including health education; immunization; family planning; and appropriate treatment for prevalent illnesses such as pneumonia, malnutrition, and sexually transmitted diseases (Carlson, 2007). Most causes of poor health and death in Ethiopia can be prevented or treated through basic methods that do not require advanced professional education. The EPHTI began about 10 years ago as an experiment in how to build a sub-Saharan country's capacity to train its own health workers, because the health challenges in Ethiopia are staggering. Consider the following figures:

- 1/6 of Ethiopian children die before age 5
- 1/2 of Ethiopian children are malnourished
- 1/8 of all Ethiopians face acute hunger
- 3/4 of Ethiopians do not have safe drinking water
- 2/5 of Ethiopians do not receive any health care whatsoever
- When the EPHTI started, life expectancy was as low as 41 years. Now, life expectancy has improved to nearly 56 years.

These realities are a challenge for Ethiopia's health care system. Tragically, most of the common illnesses and deaths that occur could be easily prevented or treated, and 10 years ago there simply were not enough health personnel to treat the mostly rural residents of this country of more than 75 million. However, while struggling under the crushing weight of poverty and killer diseases, Ethiopia has proven it can build a sustainable health workforce to meet the needs of its population through the work of the EPHTI.

This achievement is due in large part to a network of Ethiopian government officials and university faculty who have painstakingly tailored health science curricula to specifically address the Ethiopian context. These supplementary health learning materials have strengthened the education of thousands of local health workers, which has translated into improved health care delivery for approximately 56 million Ethiopians.

On the basis of a response to the expressed needs of the Ethiopia government to The Carter Center, the EPHTI was developed to address the gaps in health care at the time of Prime Minister Meles Zenawi's assumption of power in 1991. A review of the social services in Ethiopia at this time concluded that extending basic health services to the half of the Ethiopian population that was without access to basic health care was of the highest priority (Carlson, 2007). It became clear that to accomplish these objectives major changes in training mid-level and rural health workers were essential, and building a standardized preservice educational system for health care workers that could produce better quality and higher quantities of these professionals was a priority. In addition, this training had to be done in a sustainable and capacity-building way, using locally available resources, and be tailored to the Ethiopian environment.

The evolution of governmental will, international donor and nongovernmental organizational support, and grassroots participation from universities and instructors became today's EPHTI. All stakeholders from these sectors of the Ethiopian health care landscape were invited to participate in the early planning and development of the EPHTI, and a comprehensive and collaborative network was formed. Because The Carter Center planned from the beginning that the EPHTI would be locally owned and administered by Ethiopians after the initial 13-year start-up period, the resulting Ethiopian-owned initiative is one that has built the capacity of the Ethiopian health education network in a sustainable way. All the training and learning activities by the EPHTI were conducted within Ethiopian borders, and the focus on training of instructors and students was intended for the development of rural services, the premise being that people who came from rural areas will be more likely to return to rural areas to work—a theory later shown to be substantiated by Serneels et al. (2010).

The underlying principle of the EPHTI is a capacity-building strategy built around the notion that Ethiopians should play the primary role in meeting their country's community health needs. With its Ethiopian partners, The Carter Center helped the Ethiopians implement the EPHTI with three major objectives in mind:

1. Develop health learning materials (lecture notes, teaching modules, and manuals) that address the major health problems of the country and meet the specific learning needs of health center team personnel
2. Improve the knowledge and skills of faculty and instructors in teaching through intensive 2-week teaching learning workshops on pedagogical and technical skills
3. Improve the teaching learning environments of Ethiopia health sciences classrooms by providing scientific journals, relevant textbooks, teaching aides, anatomical models, computers, and basic consumable supplies and infection prevention materials

The EPHTI sought to create environments in which senior international experts would work side by side with Ethiopian teaching staff to train health center teams and develop learning materials based on Ethiopian experiences that are directly relevant to Ethiopia's health problems. The health center staff, in turn, carried the responsibility of training and supervising all community health workers, including traditional birth attendants and community health agents. Thus, the basic training for health center teams given in the universities of the EPHTI network has a direct and immediate impact on all modern primary health services throughout the country, extending even into villages and homes.

The EPHTI's interdisciplinary network of education professionals, government agencies, and practitioners takes a grassroots approach to training the next generation of Ethiopian health care workers. A fundamental tenet of the program is that Ethiopians know best how to deal with Ethiopian health issues. Thus, the focus of the program is to integrate all Ethiopian expertise—from university instructors to the female village caretakers—into specific curricula and training approaches for students studying to be health care providers. Such improved health education and training for those who treat the community—particularly women, who are not only traditional village-level health care providers but increasingly are earning more advanced degrees as clinic and hospital practitioners—benefit all levels of society through improved health. EPHTI curricula are used to train health officers (mid-level providers who are the team leaders in health clinics), nurses, female village health workers, and other specialized types of health professionals.

For more than 13 years, the EPHTI addressed the health professional train-ing challenges of Ethiopia and worked with the country's government and seven universities to develop contextualized health education materials to strengthen the training of the country's health workforce. By making these materials globally avail-able at no cost online (http://cartercenter.org/health/ephti/learning_materials/index.html), the program will be able to collaborate with government officials and university faculty of other countries to adapt a similar grassroots approach to strengthen the teaching capacities of their health professional training institutions.

Directly relevant to the country's health practices and priorities, EPHTI health learning materials are an outstanding example of how a country can tailor preservice training to meet its unique health situation. EPHTI learning materials are written by Ethiopians, for Ethiopians, and cover a wide range of topics, such as malaria, HIV/AIDS, research methodology, psychiatric nursing, and vector and rodent control. Teachers and professors at seven Ethiopian universities par-ticipated in the development of these materials and now share them across the country to educate health students, who work in primary health care centers.

The cycle of improved learning comes full circle from the student in the classroom to the women, children, and citizens in rural villages who receive that student's services on graduation. When better trained health care professionals not only provide better quality training to the community but also train and man-age future generations of community health workers, the quality and quantity of Ethiopia's health workers are increased. Not only has Ethiopia produced better educated health professionals, but also the efficiencies and grassroots approach of the EPHTI's networks have helped produce *more* of these better educated health professionals. Thus, with more health workers stationed throughout the country, parents will no longer have to trek 4 or more hours with their sick children to the closest health facility. Disease prevention can be implemented during community checkups by the 30,000 female village health-extension workers the government is now training in most remote villages. Long-term disability can be avoided with community and village surveillance and intervention from new health clinics. In short, Ethiopians' health has been improved through the work of the EPHTI, which helps Ethiopians train and educate their next generation of health workers.

ACCOMPLISHMENTS OF THE ETHIOPIA PUBLIC HEALTH TRAINING INITIATIVE

At the time this book is being written, Ethiopia has completed 8 instruction manuals, 69 training modules, and 151 sets of classroom lecture notes for use by instructors in health sciences classrooms. These 228 pieces of health learning material, which were written and customized for the Ethiopian environment, are designed to address health challenges in low-resource settings and are avail-able for free download on The Carter Center's Web site (http://cartercenter.org/health/ephti/learning_materials/index.html). In this way, the EPHTI is a model not just for Ethiopia but across the globe, for any low-resource setting.

So what has the EPHTI accomplished toward its goal of training better health workers and giving better health care to the citizens of Ethiopia? In short, it has improved the teaching of health professors and the learning environments of their students. Approximately 26,000 health center team professionals have been trained by the seven EPHTI-networked universities since its inception. These professionals have dispersed throughout the country to staff rural and urban clinics, hospitals, and health care sites and have gone on to improve the quality of health care delivered to their respective communities.

Specifically, the EPHTI has made great strides toward fulfilling the particulars of providing better health education for its students:

- Ethiopian-specific learning materials have been developed by Ethiopian faculty on almost 200 topics and in various formats, and more than 500,000 copies of these learning materials have been distributed to universities and clinics nationwide.
- More than 2,500 instructors have been trained in various skills to improve their teaching abilities.
- More than 7,000 textbooks and medical journals, and more than $500,000 in computer and laboratory equipment and teaching aids, have been given to Ethiopia's classrooms to provide better learning environments for its health students.

TEACHING LEARNING WORKSHOPS

The strengthening of Ethiopian teaching staff emerged as one of the top priorities of the EPHTI during its initial development, and addressing the needs of seven regional universities that were in turn charged with educating and training thousands of health professionals required a national comprehensive approach.

The method by which the EPHTI brought together Ethiopian health sciences faculty to meet its objective of strengthening their ability to teach was done through national teaching learning workshops. Thirteen of these 2-week workshops were held over the last 10 years of the initiative. These intensive training sessions were instrumental in meeting this primary goal of the program and, ultimately, to improve the skills of health sciences instructors in a cohesive, comprehensive, and standardized method.

Two types of national-level workshops were held: (a) one for the more senior faculty at each of the universities and (b) a general one designed for the junior faculty. The deans or administrators of the seven universities in the EPHTI network would select four senior-level faculty participants and four junior-level faculty participants to attend each annual national teaching learning workshop, for a total of 28 to 30 participants at each. After participating in the national teaching learning workshops, each group would return to their home institutions and conduct their own version of the workshops. These "cascade workshops" helped the skill strengthening techniques reach thousands of Ethiopian faculty throughout the decade of the EPHTI (see "CASCADE WORKSHOPS" section).

Each teaching learning workshop covered the topics outlined in this book, including classroom and clinical setting teaching strategies, theories of learning, understanding the learner, and evaluation. Every workshop included group discussion, field trips, and many learning activities, which are also presented in this book at the end of their corresponding chapter. All national and cascade teaching learning workshops ended with a Teaching Learning Episode (TLE), which we discuss in detail in the next section.

THE TEACHING LEARNING EPISODE

The culminating assignment for each 2-week teaching learning workshop in pedagogical skills was the presentation of a TLE. During the first week, all workshop participants were assigned to a TLE group. The two criteria for the group assignments were (a) representation of participants whose university or health facility teaching responsibilities included one or more of the disciplines in the community health team (professional nurse, health officer, medical laboratory technician, and environmental health technician) and (b) representation from at least three universities. Each group had four or five members. Each presentation was planned to last approximately 75 minutes.

Teaching Learning Episode Goals and Expectations

The teaching learning goals were discussed with the participants during the first week, with ample opportunity provided for questions and comments. The purposes of the TLE included the following:

- Provide an opportunity for faculty from the various universities to get to know each other.
- Encourage faculty to build a teaching learning network of faculty throughout the country.
- Become familiar with the modules and lecture notes, which were developed by faculty from the seven participating universities on the basis of the 30 major health problems identified by the EPHTI council. Examples of the major health problems include malaria, tuberculosis, diarrheal diseases, harmful traditional health practices, family planning, iron-deficiency anemia, and intestinal parasitosis.
- Give participants the opportunity to work together as a teaching team, assisting and learning from each other.
- Divide the assignment among the four or five members in a manner that fit the content and timeframe.
- Use a format that included learner outcomes, content, timeframe, teaching strategies, and visual aids.

These goals and expectations were shared with the participants during the early part of the workshop so that the teaching team and participants could learn from each other about the meanings conveyed by the TLE assignment.

Teaching Learning Episode Process

A class session was devoted to discussion of the steps involved in planning, developing, and evaluating a presentation. Learning Activity 10.1, at the end of this chapter, was used to guide the participants in developing their TLE. The first task was to choose a topic for the presentation. The teaching team prepared a list of about 15 of the 30 health problems identified by the EPHTI council for which there were modules and lecture notes that could be used as resource materials. We also wanted the participants to become familiar with these teaching learning resources so that they would more readily use them when they returned to their universities. Second, each group needed to decide on the educational level of students or participants they would be teaching and the location of the session, such as in a university class, at a community health center, or in a village. Because the presentation was to be given to the workshop attendees, they became the students/participants according to the designation by the TLE group presenting at the time. Third, the TLE group needed to divide the content among the group members, because all members were expected to do a part of the teaching using active teaching learning activities. After the content was divided, each group member needed to determine the learner outcomes, timeframe for each content section, appropriate teaching strategies, and visual aids.

The TLE groups were encouraged to be creative in all aspects of the teaching learning process. Supplies such as transparencies, flipcharts, pens, reading resources, and assistance with PowerPoint were available. The teaching team members also were available to meet for consultation as requested. Throughout the preparation time for the presentations, the participants were encouraged to use some of the active teaching learning strategies that had been introduced in the workshop.

Teaching Learning Episode Evaluation

There were two types of TLE evaluation: (a) peer and teaching team and (b) self-evaluation. Evaluation criteria were distributed at the outset of the assignment, in keeping with the recommendation that students and teachers should work together to understand the goals and expectations for the practice teaching sessions (Table 10.1).

Evaluation forms were distributed to all participants with written instructions about how to use a rating scale of 1 to 5 on which 1 represented minimum achievement and 5 represented maximum achievement. They were also invited to add descriptive evaluation comments for each criterion. When all of the presentations were completed, the teaching team led a general evaluation discussion, giving comments regarding all the groups. Participants were encouraged to think about the evaluation criteria for teaching and learning while listening to the presentations so as to refine and further develop their own evaluation skills.

For the presenters, emphasis was placed on the development of self-evaluation skills. To enhance this part of the evaluation process, the TLEs were videotaped.

TABLE 10.1	
EVALUATION CRITERIA FOR A TEACHING LEARNING EPISODE	
Category	**Criterion Descriptors**
Content	Appropriate to level of learner and cultural variation in the audience
Communication	Faces learners when speaking, voice is modulated, uses gestures that are culturally acceptable and appropriate, attempts to minimize vocalized pauses
Interaction with audience	Invites questions and comments, listens to learners, encourages learner-to-learner interaction
Teaching learning strategies	Uses varied active teaching learning strategies, explains the teaching learning strategies, engages learners in critical thinking
Use of media	Appropriate use of color and print, writing or print is legible
Use of time	Involves all group members, abides by time limits of the session

Each person was given a videotape of his or her TLE group's presentation with a guide for using the videotape for self-evaluation. During the preparation session we discussed how to use the videotape for self-evaluation. Participants were provided with access to Davis's (1993) book *Tools for Teaching*, with special emphasis on chapter 42, "Watching Yourself on Videotape." We also suggested that they consider asking a trusted fellow faculty member at their university to view the tape together and assist with the self-evaluation process. Davis (2009) emphasized that "faculty members at all levels and in all disciplines can benefit from the opportunity for self-reflection provided by carefully planned observation by peers or a faculty development specialist" (p. 472).

CASCADE WORKSHOPS

On the basis of the train-the-trainer concept, whereby a small set of people are trained in a subject and then those who have been trained go on to conduct their own training sessions for a larger group of people, the teaching learning workshops of the EPHTI allowed for the formation of intensive 2-week pedagogical training workshops for selected Ethiopian faculty from each university, who would then return to their respective home campuses and conduct similar intensive workshops for their colleagues. This cascade effect of pedagogical training, in 2-week workshops both at the national level and on participants' respective home campuses, was the method by which the active teaching learning strategies described in this book were utilized and disseminated.

In every cycle of the teaching learning workshops, the participants varied in seniority and pedagogical skill level. The participants of the national workshops varied every year, so that the maximum number of instructors could receive both the primary (national-level) and secondary (cascade workshop at their home institution) training. Returning to their home universities to conduct their own workshops, it was in this way that one 2-week workshop conducted each year could influence the standardized and effective skill strengthening of hundreds of Ethiopian faculty every academic calendar year. We intend that others, using this book as a guide, can replicate these teaching learning strategies and workshops in their respective teaching environments.

OTHER PROGRAMS OF THE ETHIOPIA PUBLIC HEALTH TRAINING INITIATIVE

The Health Extension Worker Program

In 2003, the Ethiopian Federal Ministry of Health launched a new comprehensive health services plan called the *Health Extension Program* (HEP; Tibebe, 2005). The HEP was designed to address the large gap between preventive and curative health needs and health services available in rural Ethiopia. It focuses on the improvement of prevention skills and behaviors within the household and thus involves fewer facility based services. Most of the activities listed in the Ethiopian government's National Health Sector Program strategies are to be implemented through the HEP.

New groups of health extension workers (HEWs) operating at the village level are the implementers of the HEP. The government of Ethiopia planned to train 30,000 HEWs within 7 years of beginning the program and is currently on track to reach that target. Training of the HEWs took place 1 year ahead of schedule thanks to the adaptation of the EPHTI curriculum for the HEWs. All HEWs were to be women, at least 18 years of age, have a minimum of a 10th-grade education, and selected by the communities in which they will work. HEWs must complete a 1-year course of instruction and field training, provided by the Ministry of Education. On completion of training, HEWs are assigned in pairs to villages where they staff health posts and work directly with individual families. As a preventive health program, the HEP promotes four areas of care: (a) disease prevention and control, (b) family health, (c) hygiene and environmental sanitation, and (d) health education and communication (Tibebe, 2005). HEWs spend 75% of their time visiting families in their homes and performing outreach activities in the community (Wilder, 2008). The remaining 25% of an HEW's time is spent providing services at health posts. HEWs are also trained to provide first aid; treat malaria, dysentery, intestinal parasites, and other ailments; and to refer cases to the nearest health center when more complicated care is needed (Wilder, 2008).

The Accelerated Health Officer Training Program

In 2005, working closely with Ethiopia's Ministry of Education, Ministry of Health, regional health bureaus, and seven partner universities, the EPHTI helped launch the Accelerated Health Officer Training Program (AHOTP), to respond to the staffing shortage caused by the growing number of new government-built community health centers in the country (Ethiopian Ministry of Health and Ministry of Education, 2005). To help jump-start the program, the EPHTI supported renovations to expand the teaching capacity of 17 training hospitals, building classrooms and libraries at these health facilities for practical training purposes. The EPHTI's curriculum, developed for regional health science universities, was also available for use in the AHOTP program. In fact, because of the existence of the EPHTI and its network of universities, the Ministry of Health was able to adapt the public health curriculum from the EPHTI health learning materials for use in the AHOTP program and was thus able to launch the ambitious AHOTP program a full year ahead of schedule.

The AHOTP program's objective is to train 5,000 health officers within 5 to 6 years (allowing for various challenges faced along the way). These newly trained health officers will be drawn from a combination of nurses and general science students, on similar tracks to upgrade their clinical skills to those of health officers.

Health officers are the leaders of the community-based health center professional staff in Ethiopia and are supported by nurses, medical laboratory technicians, environmental laboratory technicians, and health extension workers at the health center level. There is currently a shortage of health officers in Ethiopia as the government builds more health centers to serve the population's needs. The EPHTI has utilized its network of universities, the universities' affiliated training hospitals and regional health bureaus, and its health learning materials to facilitate this program.

REPLICATION OF THE ETHIOPIA PUBLIC HEALTH TRAINING INITIATIVE MODEL

With similar problems and resources, other African countries could benefit from adopting and customizing the EPHTI model for use in their national programs. The EPHTI model has been used to join universities and health professionals to explore ways to improve the education of health workers. Explorations of how to address the shortages led to universities, health centers, and hospitals working together.

In 2007, The Carter Center sponsored a replication conference in Addis Ababa, Ethiopia, and invited ministers of health and ministers of education from nine African countries: (a) Benin, (b) Sudan (both the northern and southern states), (c) Uganda, (d) Kenya, (e) Ghana, (f) Nigeria, (g) Mali, and (h) Tanzania. Other attendees included the donors: U.S. Agency for International Development, The David and Lucile Packard Foundation, The Susan Buffett Thompson Foundation, the Irish government, and others. The purpose of the replication conference was to encourage other countries to explore the possibility of replicating the EPHTI in their country. Two countries are currently seeking to implement projects similar to the EPHTI that would include the 2-week teaching learning workshops for strengthening the pedagogical skills of university instructors.

The replication conference showcased the challenges, successes, history, and methods of the initiative. As an adaptable model, even in microcosm, both in the teaching learning strategies described throughout this book and in the structure of the university network and communication process of the initiative, a program such as the EPHTI could be beneficial for other low-resource environments that seek to train quality health professionals for their underserved populations.

LEARNING ACTIVITY 10.1

DEVELOPING A TEACHING PLAN FOR A TEACHING LEARNING EPISODE

OVERVIEW

The question to be addressed in this learning activity is the following: How do we structure learning so that we address the learner at the appropriate level, know the intent of the learning, and can plan for effective evaluation?

DIRECTIONS

In this learning activity, you will be divided into groups that are, we hope, representative of the community-based team—health officer, public health nurse, medical laboratory technician, and environmental sanitarian. Each team will choose a topic from a list provided. As a group, you are to follow the directions and structure a teaching learning episode for a selected discipline, community, family, or village. You will have time to work together to plan your episode. Each member of the group is to participate, and each group will be videotaped. Videotapes will be provided to each individual so he or she can review and evaluate his or her own teaching performance. Feedback will be provided by peers and leaders.

Other questions to consider are the following: How do you teach students to move into communities, villages, and families? Where in their learning experiences do they do this? What are the current practices? Do students have the knowledge, skills, and attitudes that are needed to become quality health care workers? For this activity, consider the following variables:

a. Principles of community involvement
b. Community health workers
   Families
   Context, including health center, home, community, classroom, and other
     ctors in the setting

     ead chapter 42, "Watching Yourself on Videotape," in *Tools for Teaching* (Davis,
       his will help to inform you about how you can evaluate your teaching and
        areas of strengths and weaknesses.

DEVELOPING YOUR GROUP PRESENTATION

1. Describe the selected population (learners), that is, who, what, when, and where you teach.
   a. What level students do you teach?
2. Briefly describe the topic that your group will be teaching.
3. List three to five learning outcomes or behaviors for this teaching episode.
   a. Describe the level of learning intended for the students.
4. Describe the sources of information that you use. Use the modules, lecture notes, and other materials that you might have available.
5. What teaching materials are needed to support your teaching episode?
6. What teaching strategies are likely to accomplish desired outcome/results?
7. How will you evaluate learner achievement of objectives and/or outcomes?
8. How will you evaluate your effectiveness as a teacher?

REFERENCES

Carlson, D. (2007). History of the Ethiopia Public Health Training Initiative. In *Summary of Proceedings of the Ethiopia Public Health Training Initiative Replication Conference* (pp. 28–34). Retrieved from http://cartercenter.org/documents/ephti_repconfproceed.pdf

Chen, L., Evans, D., Evans, T., Sadana, R., Stilwell, B., Travis, P., . . . Zurn, P. (2006). *World Health Report 2006: Working together for health*. Geneva, Switzerland: World Health Organization.

Davis, B. G. (1993). *Tools for teaching*. San Francisco, CA: Jossey-Bass.

Davis, B. G. (2009). *Tools for teaching* (2nd ed.). San Francisco, CA: Jossey-Bass.

Ethiopian Ministry of Health and Ministry of Education. (2005). *Curriculum for generic and post-basic accelerated health officers training program*. Ethiopia: Author.

Serneels, P., Montalvo, J. G., Pettersson, G., Lievens, T., Butera, J. D., & Kidanu, A. (2010). Who wants to work in a rural health post? The role of intrinsic motivation, rural background and faith-based institutions in Ethiopia and Rwanda. *Bulletin of the World Health Organization, 88*, 342–349. doi:10.2471/BLT.09.072728

Tibebe, D. (2005). *Health Sector Development Programme 2005–2010*. Retrieved from http://www.moh.gov.et/index.php?option=com_remository&Itemid=59&func=fileinfo&id=2

Wilder, J. (2008). *Ethiopia's Health Extension Program: Pathfinder International's Support 2003–2007*. Retrieved from http://www.pathfind.org/site/DocServer/CBRHAs__HEWs_REVISED_REPRINT__2_.pdf?docID=11303

World Health Organization. (2010). *Ethiopia country report*. Retrieved from http://www.who.int/countries/eth/en/

Index

A

Accelerated Health Officer Training
    Program (AHOTP), 164
Accommodators, teaching
    strategies for, 41
Active teaching learning, 1–6
Active teaching learning strategies
    in Ethiopia, 159–165
    lecture as, 57–59
    Teaching Learning Framework, 1–8
    theories and research
        supporting, 17–27
    See also Application–theory–
        application (A-T-A) method;
        Patterns of knowing; and Training
        health care professionals
Active versus reflective learners, 42
Advanced organizer method, 39
Aesthetics, 19
Affective domain, 73, 142
Application cards technique, 58
Application–theory–application
    (A-T-A) method, 38–39
Apprenticeships, 24
Assessment. *See* Evaluation
    and assessment
Assimilators, 41
    teaching strategies for, 42
Assumptions, awareness
    of underlying, 61
Attitudes, teaching, 72–73

B

Behaviorist model, 4–5
Behavioral objectives, 4, 139, 142
Body, of lecture, 57
Bullet case, 102, 103
Briefing, debriefing, 79–80, 93, 101, 106

C

Carter Center, xi, xv, 160, 168
Cascade workshops, 166–167
Case Based Learning, 101–103
Case studies, 102–104
Case study formats, 101–103
    bullet cases, 102, 103
    fixed Choice Cases, 102, 103
    detailed case, 102, 103
    narrative case, 102, 103
Chalkboards, 80–82
Clinical interviews.
        See Unstructured interviews
Clinical setting, teaching in.
        See Teaching, in clinical setting
Cognitive domain, 70, 142
Communication skills, 71
Competencies, 129
Competency-based learning
        methods, 129–134
Conclusion, of lecture, 57
Constructivism, 22–23
Content mapping, 21, 27

Context-dependency model
of communication, 31
Convergers
teaching strategies for, 41
Conversation/purpose. *See* Interviewing
Critical thinking, 59–63
Cultural boundaries, 32
Cultural context, 7
Cultural openness, 33
Cultural self-awareness, 33
Culture
concept of, 31–32
and learning styles, 33
Culture-crossing skills
continuing development of, 33

D

Debriefing, 101
for Observation & Interviewing,
Field Trip, 94
for role play, 105
for simulation, 105–106
Deductive versus inductive
learners, 42
Design decisions, 103
Detailed case, 102, 103
Directed cases, 103
Discovery method, 39
Divergers, 41
teaching strategies for, 42
Domains
affective, 70, 73
cognitive, 70, 71
psychomotor, 70, 71

E

Education, concept of, 6
Educational levels
of students, 8
of learners, 71, 105, 106, 118
Educator. *See* Teacher
Emotions, 14
Empirical knowledge, 18–19
Empirical positivism, 18
Engagement phase, 54

Ethical knowledge.
See Moral knowledge
Ethiopia Public Health Training Initiative
(EPHTI), xii, xv, 68–69, 159–162
Accelerated Health Officer Training
Program (AHOTP), 168
accomplishments of, 162–163
Health Extension Worker
Program, 167
replication conference, 168–169
Ethno-religious cultures, 31
Evaluation and assessment
assessment to learning,
relating, 144–146
in clinical setting, 126–127
definitions, 137–138
goals, outcomes,
and objectives, 142–143
learning characteristics, 138–141
outcomes, evaluating, 146–147
principles of good evaluation, 138
test questions, 145–146
Evidence-based teaching
and learning practices, 8–10
Examination. *See* Observation
Experience and reflection, 53
Experiential learning. *See* Kolb's
experiential learning model
Exploratory interviews.
See Unstructured interviews
Extraversion versus
introversion, 37–38

F

Faculty guide and script, 106
Faculty/instructor role, 108–110
Feelings. *See* Attitudes
Felder–Silverman model, 42
Fieldwork
in health-related
disciplines, 77–78
Films and videotapes, 82–83
Fixed choice case, 102, 103
Flipcharts and chalkboards, 80–82
Formative evaluation, 126
Freire, Paulo, 20–21

G

Global versus sequential learners, 42
Goals, outcomes, and objectives,
    142–143
Guest speakers, 78–80

H

Health Extension Worker Program, 167
Hope, Anne, 21
Human science model, of learning, 4–5
    versus behaviorist model, 5

I

In-depth interviews. *See* Unstructured
    interviews
Inductive versus deductive learners, 42
Information versus knowledge, 68
Inquiry methods, 61–62
Instructional media and technology,
    80–84
Intellectual path, 14
Interactive teaching learning strategies, 99
    case study formats, 102–104
    classroom-based, 100
    general rules, 100–101
    problem based learning, iterative
        process of, 100
    problem-based learning (PBL), 106–110
    role play, 103–105
    service–learning, 110–117
    simulation, 105–106
Interdisciplinary panel of experts
    on teaching, learning,
        and mentoring, 79–80
Interpersonal knowledge.
        See Personal knowledge
Interviewing, 73–77
Introduction, of lecture, 56–57
Introversion versus extraversion, 37
    teaching strategies for, 38
Intuition versus sensing. *See* Sensing
        versus intuition
I–Thou encounter, 19

J

Judging versus perceptive
    people, 40–41
Judgments and decisions making, 63

K

Kindezi method, of East Africa, 34
Knowledge
    development of, 18
    versus information, 68
    teaching, 70–71
Kolb learning cycle model, 41–42
Kolb's experiential learning
    model, 23
KSA (knowledge, skills, and
    attitudes), 70

L

Laudun, Larry, 18
Leadership theories and competencies,
    151–152
    fundamental practices, 152–155
Learners, understanding, 29–48
Learning
    behaviorist model of, 4
    characteristics of, 138–141
    concept of, 4–5
    facilitating, 125–126
    human science model of, 4
    levels of theory and, 140–141
    teaching intent, 139–140
Learning activities
    case studies, problem-based learning,
        simulation, or role play, developing
        case for, 118
    clarifying definitions, 11–15
    critical thinking, 65
    culture and learning, 44–48
    field trip to health center for
        observation and interview
        assignment, 93–95
    interdisciplinary panel, on teaching,
        learning, and mentoring, 96

Learning activities (*cont.*)
  learning styles, 48
  observation and interviewing, in
    health centers and hospitals,
    91–95
  personal and professional leadership
    activities, developing, 156
  service-learning experience, developing,
    119–120
  sources of information overview, 85
  teaching knowledge, skills, and
    attitudes, 86–90
  teaching plan for teaching learning
    episode, developing, 170–171
  test questions, developing, 148
  using instructional media
    and technology, 97
  using storytelling and reflection
    in lectures, 64
  ways of knowing, 25–27
Learning experience, in health-related
    disciplines, 77–78
Learning styles, 35–43
Learning Styles Inventory (LSI), 41
Learning theory, 22–24
Lectures, 55–59
Life ways, cultural, 31
Lifelong commitment, to cultural
    openness, 33
Low-resource environments, 159–165
  Objectives: SMART objectives,
    106, 118

M

Mastery learning, 130
  cycle for, 133, 134
Matching questions, 146
Meaning, assigning, 62–63
Metaphor and symbols recognition, 63
Mini-cases, 102
Model, concept of, 22
Moral knowledge, 20
Multiple-choice questions, 145
  examples in, 147
Myers–Briggs Type Indicator (MBTI),
    37–41

N

Narrative case, 102, 103
Nominal Group Method, 38, 39, 40
Nonparticipant observation, 74, 75
  steps in, 75–76
Nonstructured interviews, 74

O

Observation, 73–76
Observed Structured Clinical Examination
    (OSCE), 144
One-Minute Preceptor model, 127–128

P

Paradigm shift, 5
Paraphrasing, 58
Participant observation, 74
Participatory education, 20–21
Passive versus active learning, 138
Pattern recognition, 62
Patterns of knowing, 18–20
Perception knowledge.
    See Aesthetics
Perceptive versus judging
    people, 40
  teaching strategies for, 40–41
Personal knowledge, 19
Philosophical bases, for teaching and
    learning, 2–6
PowerPoint presentations, 84
Preparation, in clinical setting
  curriculum, knowing, 123–124
  learner, knowing, 124
  site, knowing, 124–125
Preparation phase, 54
Problem-based learning (PBL), 107–110
Processing phase, 54
Projectors and transparencies, 82
Psychomotor skill, 71

Q

Questioning, 62

R

Reflection, for learning, 52–55
Reflective thinking.
      See Critical thinking
Reflective versus active learners, 42
Role play, 103–105

S

Scientific revolutions, 5
Script and faculty guide, 106
Self-directed learning model, 125
Sensing versus intuition, 38–39
   Felder–Silverman learning styles
      model, 42
Sequential versus global learners, 42
Service–Learning, 110–117
Short answer/essay questions, 146
Short writes, 58
Silence, 34
Simulation, 105–107
Situational learning, 23–24
Skillful teaching, 4
Skinner, B. F., 4
Small group work, strategies to
      facilitating, 59
SMART objectives, 106
SNAPPS (**S**ummarize, **N**arrow
      possibilities, **A**nalyze, **P**robe,
      Plan, and **S**elect), 128–134
Sources of information, 67–69
Spirituality, 14
Storytelling, 51–52
   and reflection, 55
Structured interviews, 74
Superior leadership, 152
Symbols recognition, 63

T

Task analysis process, 71, 129,
      131–132
Teacher
   challenging the process,
      152–153

enabling others to act, 154–155
encouraging the heart, 155
as leader, role model, and mentor,
      151–156
leadership theories
      and competencies, 151–152
modeling the way, 155
preparing for, 14
role of, 10
shared vision, inspiring, 153–154
Teaching
   attitudes, 72–73
   concept of, 3–4
   fieldwork, learning experience in
      health-related disciplines, 77–78
   implications for, 43
   knowledge, 70–71
   observation and interviewing, 73–77
   skills, 71–72
   sources of information overview,
      67–69
   tools for, 67–84
   using guest speakers, 78–80
   using instructional media
      and technology, 80–84
Teaching and learning context,
      in low-resource countries, 6–7
   in classroom, 7–8
Teaching, in classroom settings, 51–63
Teaching, in clinical setting, 123–134
Teaching, intent of
   strategies for identifying, 139–140
   students learning, 139
Teaching learning episode
      (TLE), 164–166
Teaching Learning Framework, 1–8
Teaching learning workshops,
      167–168
Technology. *See* Instructional media and
      technology
Test questions, writing and evaluating,
      163–164
Think Aloud Paired Problem Solving
      (TAPPS), 38, 39, 40, 58–59
Thinking versus feeling, 39–40
Think–Pair–Share, learning strategy,
      11, 13, 58

Timmel, Sally, 21
Training, concept of, 6
Training health care professionals
 Accelerated Health Officer Training
  Program (AHOTP), 168
 cascade workshops, 166–167
 Ethiopia Public Health Training
  Initiative (EPHTI), 159–163,
  168–169
 Health Extension Worker
  Program, 167
 in low-resource environments,
  159–171
Training health care professionals (*cont.*)
 teaching learning episode (TLE),
  164–166
 teaching learning workshops,
  163–164
Transcultural skills. *See* Culture-crossing
 skills
Transformational leadership, 152
Transparencies. 82–83

True–false questions, 146
Tutor role, 108

U

Unstructured interviews, 76–77

V

Verbal versus visual learners, 42
Videotapes and films, 82–83
Visual versus verbal learners, 42

W

Western and non-western cultures
 and education, 29–30
What must be known (WMBK) method,
 38, 71
Why method. *See* Discovery method